DR. PAULA MOYNAHAN'S

COSMETIC SURGERY FOR WOMEN

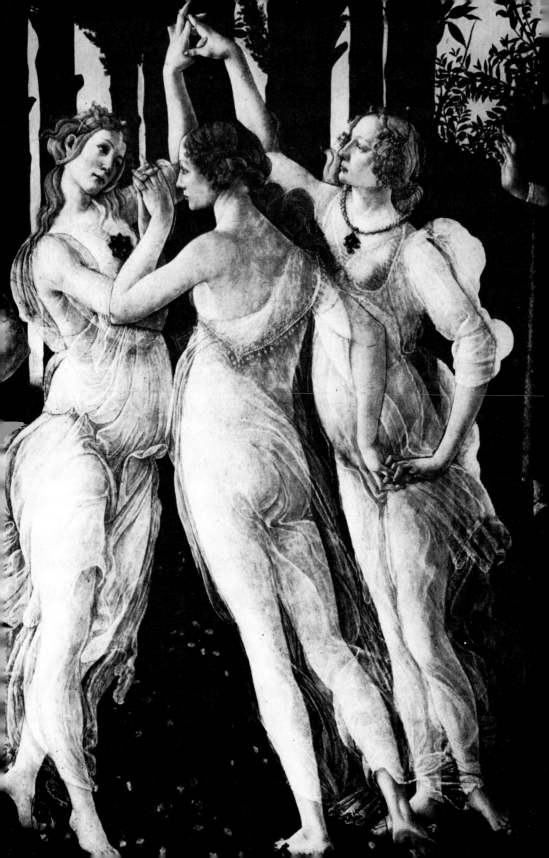

DR. PAULA MOYNAHAN'S

COSMETIC SURGERY FOR WOMEN

Paula A. Moynahan, M.D.

A Revolutionary Approach to Image Enhancement

Crown Publishers, Inc. / New York

Publisher's Note: This book contains case histories derived from interviews and research. The relevant facts have not been altered. However, names and other identifying details have been changed. While the book discusses certain issues, situations, and choices regarding cosmetic surgery, it is not intended as a substitute for professional medical advice.

Published by Crown Publishers, Inc., 225 Park Avenue South, New York, New York 10003, and represented in Canada by the Canadian MANDA Group

CROWN is a trademark of Crown Publishers, Inc.

Manufactured in the United States of America

Library of Congress Cataloging-in-Publication Data

Moynahan, Paula A.
    Dr. Paula Moynahan's cosmetic surgery for women.

    1. Surgery, Plastic.   2. Women — Surgery.
I. Title.   II. Title: Cosmetic surgery for women.
III. Title: Doctor Paula Moynahan's cosmetic surgery for
women.   [DNLM: 1. Surgery, Plastic — popular works.
WO 600 M938c]
RD119.M69   1988   617'.95   87-15541
ISBN 0-517-56429-7

Book design by June Marie Bennett

10   9   8   7   6   5   4   3   2   1

First Edition

To my parents,
Brunilda and Paul Moynahan,
and my brother,
Timothy Constant Moynahan

CONTENTS

PREFACE

*I am the beauty of woman . . . You
will find my likeness in the radiancy
of flowers, in the grace of the palm
trees; in the flight of pigeons, in the
bound of the gazelle, in the rippling
of brooks, in the soft light of the
moon; and if you close your eyes,
you will find me within yourself.*

ANATOLE FRANCE, *Thais*

eauty. As a plastic surgeon, I deal daily with people who come to me hoping to capture this elusive ideal, a quest as old as humankind.

An exact definition of beauty has eluded both poets and philosophers. Part of the reason is that the image of ideal beauty as expressed in art and literature has changed from one people to another and one generation to the next.

The Kirghiz people, a Monogolian tribe, once believed that their race presented the ultimate in human beauty because their facial bone structure resembled that of the horse, to them the sublime masterpiece of all creation.

The Greek ideal of a physically perfect form, as seen in the statues of sculptors like Phidias and Praxiteles, has dominated Western ideas of beauty. It was reborn during the Renaissance and has influenced us ever since, even accounting for some of the qualities that distinguished early Hollywood beauties such as Marlene Dietrich or Joan Crawford. One photographer said of Crawford in 1970, "By strength of purpose and her own design, [she] created a face with the architectural qualities of a head sculptured by Phidias. Her bone structure was the delight of cameramen, painters, and sculptors."

Today we know that the perfect oval face considered the ideal for so long actually ages more rapidly than its less perfect sister, while faces with less regular features grow more interesting with age. We still value the classic ideal but allow for more individual standards of beauty. Art historian Kenneth Clark summed up the dual standard most common in our time when he wrote, "'Classic' beauty, which reached its climax in ancient Greece, depends on symmetry, established proportion, and regular features. 'Characteristic' beauty treats the features with greater freedom and will allow a *retroussé* (turned up) nose and small sparkling eyes, provided they give the face greater animation."

With this new freedom of individuality, anthropologist Desmond Morris has observed that it is not necessarily standards of beauty that change, but rather beautiful women who "insist upon changing shape" from society to society. "To one culture, it is vitally important that a girl should be extremely plump; to another it is essential that she should be slender and willowy; to yet another she must have an hourglass shape with a tiny waist," Morris noted.

As a cosmetic surgeon I know that the standards of beauty set by society are vital influences on the self-image of my patients. I also know that each woman's goals must be based on her own reality and should not follow an arbitrary ideal or the idea that surgery can transform you into something totally different from your own form.

Plastic surgery is not magic. No surgical procedure can restore lost youth or turn a fifty-year-old face into that of a twenty-year-old. Cosmetic surgery will not save a failing marriage or bring back a lost love, and changing a single feature will not transform you into a movie star. There is little point in having a Grace Kelly nose with a Gene Kelly chin or ears!

What surgery can do is to correct problems and enhance your own individual look, giving a cleaner, younger, and more refreshed appearance that can help you to like yourself better and feel more self-confident. It can give a lift to the inner self as well as the outer image.

It is this opportunity to help the whole person that attracted me to my profession. I made the decision to become a physician when I was still a young child, encouraged by my father to find a field that would both help people and help me to make my place in the world. It was an unlikely decision for a little girl going to a two-room school in rural Connecticut, and when I announced to my second-grade teacher that I planned to become a doctor, she called the principal in to hear the news. Both of these women encouraged me and celebrated my medical school graduation with me. Their presence was a source of great pride to me as well as to them.

It was my sixth-grade teacher who suggested that I attend a women's college, the College of Mount Saint Vincent, where my aspirations would be further encouraged. Afterward, I chose the Women's Medical College in Philadelphia, at that time the only school in the Western Hemisphere dedicated solely to medical education for women, an environment that allowed me to pursue my education without experiencing the discrimination women doctors were subjected to not so many years ago. It seems incredible with today's medical school classes almost half female that only eighteen years ago women comprised just 3 percent of all physicians in the United States.

I was attracted immediately to surgery because it suited my personality; it enabled me to use my hands and to see instant good results from my efforts. It was during my surgery residency at Lenox Hill Hospital in New York City that I was first exposed to plastic surgery and the special benefits it could bring. It was a way to help my patients achieve the Greek ideal of health in both mind and body, to offer improvement to the inner spirit by changing the outer shell, and I decided it was worth the extra years of study to devote myself to this task.

Once again, it was an unusual decision for a woman. In 1975 when I completed the seven years of training required to become board certified in both general and plastic surgery, there were only sixteen American women in the world that were certified by the American Board of Plastic Surgery. Happily, the number is growing as more women seek medical careers, but even today only 3 percent of the twenty-eight hundred plastic surgeons with board certification are female.

Some plastic surgeons devote their major energies to performing reconstructive procedures, correcting disfigurements or malformations resulting from birth defects, disease, burns, accidents, or other trauma. Though many of the surgical procedures I perform are reconstructive in nature, as a cosmetic surgeon I deal primarily with patients who have chosen to undergo surgery expressly to improve their appearance. I enjoy this branch of surgery because of its positive effect on patients and because of the artistic satisfaction it affords me.

While the numbers of men seeking the benefits of cosmetic surgery are growing dramatically, the great majority of those who elect to enhance their looks through surgery are women, and my own practice is almost 75 percent female. Thus, while one of the chapters to come will be devoted to men, this is primarily a woman surgeon's book to women, reflecting the special concerns I hear expressed everyday in my practice and that I understand.

The striving to attain an image of beauty is held up as a feminine ideal from our earliest years. While standards of what is considered beautiful may change, one element remains constant for women. As expressed by philosopher Thomas Hobbes in seventeenth-century England, again a century later by French writer Stendahl, and by American historian Will Durant in our own century, beauty for women has been allied to a promise of happiness or pleasure—often associated with an erotic pleasure. Because so much of a woman's sexual identity is tied to her appearance, a marked defect or the inevitable lessening of youthful beauty caused by aging has special significance for the female psyche. This is heightened as a woman approaches mid-life because the changes in the face and body brought on by menopause are more rapid and concentrated than the gradual changes experienced by men as they age.

Cosmetic surgery is not a painless panacea that restores lost youth. It cannot radically change your image or your life and it may not be right for everyone.

However, cosmetic surgery has enabled many women to face the world more confidently by correcting defects that have made them self-conscious and by softening the harsh effects of aging. It allows you to be the best you can be for as long as you possibly can, to come as close as you can to your own ideal beauty. It is still a relative luxury, but one that more and more people can afford. Today, my patients come from every walk of life and many of them are simply foregoing or deferring a vacation to spend their money on something more lasting in its rewards.

My hope is to educate you to the exciting possibilities of today's cosmetic surgery, to give you the realistic knowledge you need to understand what it can and cannot do for you, to decide whether it is right for you, and, if so, to proceed with peace of mind.

May the results enable your mirror, your family, and your friends to apply to you the meaning of the French compliment, *Elle est bien dans sa peau* ("She lives well in her skin").

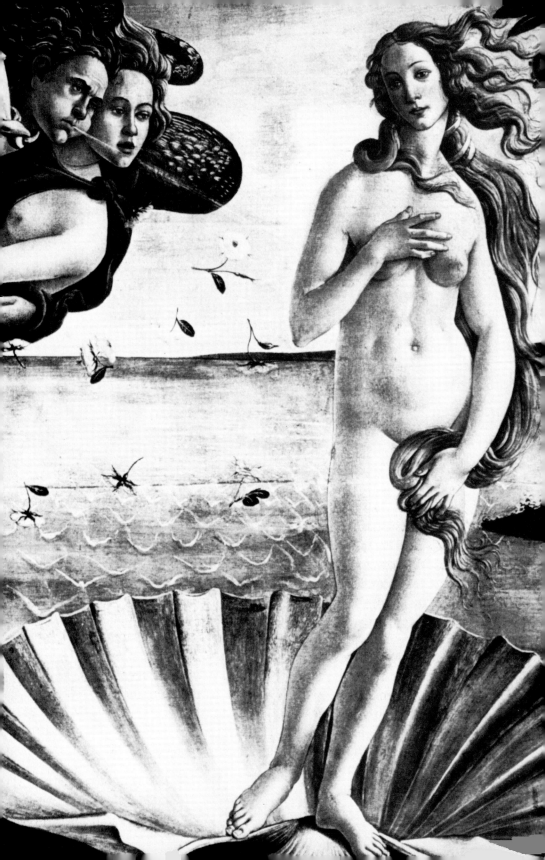

INTRODUCTION

To be born woman is to know—
Although they do not talk of it at school—
That we must labour to be beautiful.

WILLIAM BUTLER YEATS, "Adam's Curse"

osmetic surgery is an idea whose time has come.

It is not a new idea. The ancient Assyrians used ivory implants to try to create the strong hooked nose considered attractive in their society. Ancient Chinese women bound their feet to make them dainty. Many primitive peoples scarred their bodies to conform to the idea of beauty that prevailed in their own times.

But in our own times, the art of surgery to improve the appearance has reached a state of excellence never dreamed of even a generation ago. The tight mask once associated with a face-lift has been replaced by soft, naturally youthful contours. Finer stitching materials, improved techniques, and skillful placement today help conceal scars. More refined drugs allow more control and fewer complications in surgery, antibiotics have lessened the dangers of infection, and improved materials have minimized the risks of rejection when used for reconstruction.

New procedures such as lipolysis have made it possible to resculpt major portions of the body with minimal discomfort or risk. Much of this surgery today is ambulatory, done right in the doctor's office with the patient returning home the same day, which has greatly reduced the cost of surgery and made it accessible to many more people.

Attitudes have changed as dramatically as techniques. Wanting to look your best is no longer considered vanity nor is cosmetic surgery considered something to hide. First lady Betty Ford was candid about her face-lift and all America knew when first lady Nancy Reagan used a cosmetic surgeon to have a skin cancer removed from her face. Comedienne Phyllis Diller announced in the *Los Angeles Times* that she was giving a party to celebrate the fifth anniversary of her face-lift, inviting everyone who had ever had a face-lift to attend and quipping, "That ought to include at least everyone in Hollywood."

Even etiquette arbiter Amy Vanderbilt discussed her face-lift on television and Senator William Proxmire achieved instant celebrity when he continued his regular congressional duties with the not-yet-healed scars from his hair transplants plainly visible.

Cosmopolitan editor Helen Gurley Brown is one of the most enthusiastic advocates of cosmetic surgery, stating, "Over the past eighteen years I've had rhinoplasty (nose bump removed), dermabrasion (skin scraped), and my 'eyes done.' Should you do some of these major things 'after the fall'? I would *hope* so . . . how wonderful that these operations exist, have been perfected so much, and can help so much. Many beautiful women (and men) that you think look terrific after fifty have had surgery."

Once these benefits were the province of the rich and famous, but as cosmetic surgery becomes more acceptable and less expensive, the numbers who elect to have surgery each year to improve their appearance are multiplying rapidly. In 1949 about fifteen thousand Americans underwent cosmetic surgery. In 1984 a survey by the American Society of Plastic and Reconstructive Surgeons (ASPRS) showed that over seventy thousand people had surgery to change the shape of their noses alone! The total number having cosmetic surgery had risen to almost half a million—and more than half of these patients had annual incomes of twenty-five thousand dollars or less.

One reason for these growing numbers is that women seeking surgery are younger than they used to be. A recent survey showed that 43 percent of those having plastic surgery are thirty-five or younger. Ten years ago the average age of a woman seeking a face-lift was sixty; today it is fifty, and it is not uncommon to find forty-year-olds coming in for face-lifts.

Nor is it only women who are enjoying the benefits offered by cosmetic surgery. The ASPRS reported in 1986 that the number of men having cosmetic surgery had grown to 35 percent of all patients.

Many who come to see me have been thinking about having cosmetic surgery for a long time—sometimes for years. One of the strong motivations I hear is society's great emphasis today on youth and fitness. With many of us taking better care of ourselves generally, we want our bodies to keep pace with our energetic spirits. As one of my patients said to me: "I've been jogging and exercising and paying attention to nutrition. I've done all I can to get the inside of my body healthy; now it's time to do something about the outside."

Also, today's women have joined men in worrying about staying competitive in a youth-oriented job market.

Prospective patients come to me with many questions, questions you probably share. The pages ahead will answer these points, giving you the information you need on the options and the wide range of possibilities offered by today's cosmetic surgery. They will be your private first consultation, offering the same kind of accurate medical and personal information I would give you in my own office, telling you what to expect during and following each major area of cosmetic surgery, both facial surgery (face-lifts, eyelids, ear, and nose) and body contouring (breasts, abdomen, hips, thighs, buttock, and arms).

A special chapter will bring you up-to-date on recent developments in skin treatments such as collagen, chemical peel, dermabrasion, and retinoic acid, breakthroughs that are enabling many men and women to look years younger.

My aim is to give the facts and dispel the myths about a branch of surgery that is sometimes misunderstood. For while cosmetic surgeons are, indeed, performing what many consider miracles, they are surgeons, not magicians, and no surgery should be entered into lightly without a full understanding of the procedures and the possible complications involved. As with any kind of surgery, the more information you have beforehand, the happier you are likely to be with the result.

When you undertake cosmetic surgery with realistic expectations, it can give an invaluable boost to your image and your sense of self. A skilled surgeon can bring greater harmony and balance to your face and body by correcting imperfections, and help to slow (though not to stop) the march of time.

However, since all surgery holds some element of risk, the first and most important step, if you are considering a procedure to enhance your appearance, is to find a well-qualified surgeon.

CHOOSING A COSMETIC SURGEON

With the growing interest in the field, there has been a corresponding increase in the number of doctors practicing cosmetic surgery. While this increased demand has attracted many well-qualified practitioners, it also means that many surgeons vary widely in their training in cosmetic surgery today.

As with any medical specialty, the more thorough the physician's training, skill, and experience, the better your chances of a happy experience with cosmetic surgery. The choice is too important to be made on the basis of a television commercial or a tip from your beautician. Your doctor should have top professional credentials.

The American Society of Plastic and Reconstructive Surgeons (ASPRS), a group founded in 1931 to promote optimal quality care for plastic surgery patients, is conducting a nationwide campaign to educate consumers on what to look for in a doctor's credentials. Any physician is allowed to perform surgical procedures in the state in which he or she is licensed. However, of forty thousand plastic surgeons throughout the country, only twenty-eight hundred are board certified by the American Board of Plastic Surgery. To qualify for this certification, doctors must have completed four years of medical school, four or five years of general surgery training, and at least two years of training in an approved plastic surgery residency program. They must also have passed a rigorous written and oral examination. Board certification is your guarantee of proper training.

Your personal physician or a friend who has had a good experience with plastic surgery are excellent sources of referrals to competent plastic surgeons. Other places to be consulted are your local county medical society or a community hospital, particularly if it is a teaching hospital. Hospital personnel who see the surgeon in action and work with his or her patients are also good people to ask for recommendations. You can also call the American Society of Plastic and Reconstructive Surgeons for the names of qualified physicians living in your area of the country. Their toll-free number is 1-800-635-0635.

To be doubly sure of your choice, check that the surgeon is board certified when you call for an appointment. Ask your physician to check the doctor's standing in the local medical community. In the office, look for the framed certificate proving board certification. If it is not posted on the wall, ask to see it. If college diplomas are not posted, ask where the doctor was trained as well. Ethical doctors welcome questions from their patients about their qualifications and training, and you

AESTHETIC SURGICAL PROCEDURES IN 1984

PROCEDURE	PERCENT CHANGE	CASES	FEE RANGE
Breast augmentation	+32%	95,000	$1,000–3,000
Blepharoplasty (Mainly eye tucks)	+31%	73,900	$600–4,000
Rhinoplasty (Nose)	+30%	70,500	$1,000–4,500
Rhytidectomy (Face-lift; includes forehead lifts)	+39%	54,400	$1,500–8,000
Suction lipectomy (Fat removal)	N/A	55,900	$300–4,000
Dermabrasion	+38%	23,500	$250–2,500
Abdominoplasty (Tummy tuck)	+37%	20,900	$1,500–5,000
Mentoplasty (Chin implant)	+40%	17,500	$250–3,000
Mastopexy (Breast lift)	+26%	16,200	$1,000–4,000
Chemical peel	+67%	16,200	$250–2,500
Otoplasty (Ears)	+15%	13,200	$750–3,500
Hair transplantation	+7%	4,500	$300–5,000
Surgical body contour	+300%	16,000	$500–5,000

Source: American Society of Plastic and Reconstructive Surgeons

should never hesitate to verify their credentials. You should also know whether the doctor has present hospital or university affiliations, and be sure that he or she is accredited and in good standing with a reputable local hospital. It is an advantage if the surgeon practices reconstructive as well as cosmetic surgery, since one technique borrows heavily from the other.

Beware of doctors who advertise heavily. The ASPRS advertising guidelines stress educating the consumer and providing tools for the selection of a properly trained and certified surgeon, but much current advertising is not aimed to educate. It plays on the emotional appeal of cosmetic surgery without giving full facts about it as a medical procedure. Do not be tempted by this kind of message. You need a doctor who offers sound credentials, not pretty pictures.

Finally, never shop for bargain prices for surgery. It is a foolish economy not to seek the best qualified doctor you can afford.

PATIENT-DOCTOR RAPPORT

Having rapport and trust in your surgeon is especially important in so personal an area as cosmetic surgery. A doctor may have superb credentials, but if you do not feel you are communicating well, or that he or she is not taking the time to listen and answer your questions fully, then that surgeon may be wrong for you. I have occasionally heard from patients about a doctor specializing in reconstructive surgery who discourages procedures for strictly cosmetic reasons, and conversely, about doctors who try to persuade patients to sign up for more surgery than they had requested. Be wary of either approach. You and your doctor should agree on what surgery can do for you. If you are not happy with your first interview, consult other surgeons. It is worth the cost of consultation fees to find the right doctor for you.

You will want to be sure to choose a doctor who will not

abandon you after surgery. Plastic surgery should not be cut, sew, and good-bye. Make sure your doctor will be accessible in person or by phone to take care of you. If you must go through an entourage of receptionists and nurses before you get to the doctor, consider carefully whether you will be happy with the relationship.

ARE YOU A CANDIDATE FOR COSMETIC SURGERY?

One of the prime roles of a responsible surgeon is to help you determine whether you are a proper candidate for cosmetic surgery. It has been said that the ideal cosmetic surgeon must be part physician, part artist, and part psychologist, and all these facets will play a role in your initial interview.

Medical expertise comes into play as the doctor evaluates your overall physical condition, as well as the physical condition of the skin, the physical age of a patient as opposed to her chronological age, the presence or absence of fat in the area to be operated on, and the underlying bone structure. These affect the degree of correction or improvement that is possible as much as the doctor's artistic skill.

While the results of surgery are often better and longer lasting before significant aging has taken place, most surgeons won't operate until significant benefits can be achieved. For example, a procedure other than a face-lift can be recommended, such as a collagen injection or a chemical peel, if the doctor does not feel you are ready for more extensive surgery.

The doctor must gently remind prospective patients of the realities of surgery. You should understand the temporary inconvenience and physical restraints that will follow, such as swelling or discomfort. You may want to make plans for possible loss of time from work or provide for help in the care of the family during your period of recuperation. While these are short-lived results, they are facts of life for almost any type of surgery and need to be recognized before you choose elective surgery.

The surgeon's role as psychologist comes into even stronger focus when you discuss your reasons for having surgery. Cosmetic surgery, especially facial surgery, deals as much with self-image as with physical appearance. Patients usually look and feel better afterward, but those who expect the surgery to change the course of their lives are doomed to disappointment. So is any sixty-year-old who hopes to look as she did at thirty, or any patient who is having surgery done at the urging of another person, whether a friend, husband, or parent. A conscientious doctor will not operate on a patient who has unrealistic expectations. Patients who think the shape of their nose or breasts or a few wrinkles are responsible for their problems are not likely to be satisfied with the results of their surgery.

The healthiest reason I know for seeking cosmetic surgery and the one I like best to hear from a prospective patient is simply, "I want to look better and feel better about myself. My family loves me just like I am, and they are behind me, but they are not the reason I want to do this. It is strictly for myself."

THE FIRST INTERVIEW

In an initial interview both doctor and patient will be screening each other. From the doctor's point of view, the ideal candidate is someone in good general health who is highly motivated to improve her appearance and who has realistic expectations about the recuperative period and the final results of the surgery.

When you arrive for your interview, the nurse or receptionist will ask you to fill out the same kind of general health form used by any physician seeing you for the first time. You will be asked about your overall health, your previous medical history, any drug you take currently, whether you have drug or other allergies, and the reason for your visit, as well as the name of the person who referred you to the office. Based on this medical data, the doctor will be able to determine whether your general state of health is proper for surgery. Before any surgery is undertaken, a physical examination is mandatory, along with standard blood tests and urinalysis that may identify any possible complications.

The form may also ask about your reasons for wanting surgery. If you prefer to wait to discuss this privately with the doctor, simply say so.

When the doctor has reviewed your history with you, he or she will probably ask you to explain in your own words what kind of surgery you are seeking and why. The "why" is as important to the doctor as the "what." It will tell the doctor something about your personal self-image. If your hopes are unrealistic—if you are expecting surgery to cure ailing relationships, salvage a fallen career, or ensure eternal youth—you are among those contemplating surgery for the wrong reasons and a conscientious doctor will tactfully discourage you from proceeding.

The doctor may also ask about your private life, whether there has been a recent trauma such as divorce or death in the family, which might indicate emotional upset that would make a delay in surgery advisable.

While you are chatting, the doctor's practiced eye is noting your appearance and the changes you can realistically expect from surgery. You will move next into an examining room with a mirror where the surgeon will analyze with you in understandable terms the medical procedures that will be involved if you have surgery, and what the results will be. It is important that you understand just what surgery can and cannot do for you. Take your time and ask all the questions that concern you about every part of the surgical process from start to finish.

Be sure you are clear about the fees for surgery and whether any portion can be covered by insurance. Most insurance policies do not cover cosmetic surgery other than a few special cases, such as when nasal surgery is required to correct a breathing problem, or if droopy eyelids interfere with vision. Some corporations are now beginning to include plastic surgery in their executive benefits package, however, and you will find that ambulatory surgery done on an outpatient basis reduces costs considerably because no hospital stay is required. Plastic surgery costs also may be included as tax deductible medical expenses.

Ask about the risks involved in surgery as well as the benefits. You should be fully prepared for the recuperation period and for the scarring that will be left after surgery. It is not possible to cut through the full thickness of the skin without scars resulting. Part of the cosmetic surgeon's art is to hide these scars in the natural folds and creases of the face and body and behind the hairline so that they will not be noticeable. Still, even the most successful operation leaves some scars and you should know just what to expect.

PHOTOGRAPHS AND MODELS

If you and your surgeon agree that you are a candidate for cosmetic surgery, the routine next step is to schedule detailed photographs of the area to be operated on. I discuss these in depth with every patient and study them in planning her surgical procedure. Sometimes I refer to them during the procedure itself. Eventually, they become part of the permanent record as a basis for "before and after" comparisons.

You may come back as often as necessary before surgery to discuss the different aspects revealed by the camera and to decide definitely which ones you want changed.

Some doctors use photographs and sketches of patients from previous operations to help you decide how you would like to look. Some have even introduced computerized video imaging as part of the preoperative consultation, drawing a computer sketch of the "new you" after surgery.

I prefer not to use either pictorial models or *moulages* (impressions) of noses, eyes, or faces. Neither photographs, pen and ink drawings, computer imaging, nor wax or plaster molds are the same as flesh, skin, or cartilage, and models cannot always be duplicated, so I do not find this a satisfactory way to proceed. Computer images, which are two-dimensional rather than three-dimensional, have special drawbacks. Because of the significant differences in how individual tissue heals, there may be no relationship between the electronic image and the final surgical result, and patients may be disappointed.

Rather than trying to fit you to a likeness of someone else, I believe the surgeon should take account of your uniqueness and explore with you how to present your best self to the world by maximizing your personal strengths and minimizing your weaknesses.

Several years ago I had a patient whose friends told her she bore a strong resemblance to Elizabeth Taylor. She was indeed an attractive woman and she did look like the film beauty in some respects—the same dark hair, the large and beautiful violet eyes—but she had an arched nose with a slight hook at the tip that was decidedly different from her ideal. When I told her she could not expect to have Elizabeth Taylor's exact nose, she rebelled. "I want it," she insisted. No amount of persuasion could convince her that, without Miss Taylor's genetic makeup, bone structure, and skin texture, she could not expect to become an exact likeness. Finally she agreed that a nose that was similar to Elizabeth Taylor's without being an exact duplicate would satisfy her. Nevertheless, when she was wheeled into the operating room and the surgical sheets were drawn back to prepare her for surgery, I found pinned to her hospital gown a large picture of Elizabeth Taylor!

Another question that frequently comes up in the initial interview with patients involves ethnic characteristics, particularly the shape of noses and eyes. Once it was commonplace to try to erase distinct racial features, but a healthy growth in national and ethnic pride has changed this. Back in 1971, *Medical World News* was among the first to suggest that cosmetic surgeons learn how to provide African rather than Anglo-Saxon characteristics for their black patients. That same year a group of Jewish students made headlines showing their national pride in the state of Israel by proclaiming that "Jewish Is Beautiful," and urging Jews to maintain their racial identities, particularly the nose and other strong facial characteristics. Asians also are taking more pride in their characteristic features. Today a conscientious surgeon urges enhancement of these features rather than total eradication of a person's ethnic identity.

PREOPERATIVE AND POSTOPERATIVE CARE

Along with details of the surgical procedure itself, you should ask about the preoperative and postoperative care the doctor will prescribe.

Though specific directions will depend on the type of surgery being performed, your overall health should be in top form before any surgery. I recommend not smoking six weeks prior to surgery, and exercising three or four times a week to increase surface blood flow and boost immune function. I also find that vitamin C supplements begun two weeks prior to surgery and continued afterward promote quicker healing with less bruising and scar formation.

For patients scheduled for face-lifts or other facial surgery, an intensive skin care program to deep cleanse and stimulate the skin before an operation produces well-nourished and moisturized skin that makes a tremendous difference in the scar tissue formation and appearance after surgery. Following surgery, skin treatments that help reduce swelling and increase blood circulation and overall tissue tone are also beneficial. The results are so excellent that I now automatically include both preoperative and postoperative facial care as part of routine facial surgery.

If you decide on surgery, you will be given careful instructions about not eating or drinking anything after midnight preceding the following day's surgery. Equally important, you will be cautioned not to take aspirin or any aspirin-containing products for at least ten days before surgery. Because it interferes with platelet adhesiveness, the blood-clotting mechanism the body uses to stop bleeding, aspirin is not advisable before any type of surgery. One of the reasons for letting the surgeon know what medications you are using is to be sure that none of them contains aspirin.

HOSPITAL VERSUS AMBULATORY SURGERY

Ambulatory surgery—surgery that is performed in a doctor's private operating room or in a freestanding facility outside a hospital—has multiplied rapidly in recent years, helping greatly to curtail the cost of cosmetic surgery. According to the ASPRS, over 90 percent of eyelid surgery and chin implants and over 50 percent of nasal surgery and face-lifts today are done on an ambulatory or outpatient basis.

Whether your surgery will be done in an office operating room or in a hospital depends on your personal preferences and your doctor's professional judgment. A patient who is afraid might be reassured by a hospital setting. Those who live alone with no one available to care for them after surgery, or those who prefer not to have a strange nurse in the home, may opt for hospitalization as well, and some medical conditions require hospitalization. While heart ailments, hypertension, thyroid conditions, kidney disease, or diabetes are not absolute barriers to surgery, it stands to reason that people with such problems are more at risk. If any of these conditions are advanced, in fact, they may preclude surgery entirely.

When there is an option, studies have shown that patients do better both physically and psychologically when they have ambulatory surgery out of the hospital. They are already familiar with the staff taking care of them, which is reassuring. The patient-to-staff ratio is better and the staff is expert in caring for plastic surgery patients. If complications from cosmetic surgery occur, they are recognized and treated immediately. It can be true that a patient having elective surgery such as a face-lift will not receive the same attention in a busy hospital as someone in for more life-threatening surgery.

A real psychological benefit is going home the same day. Most of us just plain feel better recuperating in our beds than in a hospital room.

The precautions taken during surgery in an office operating room are the same as those in the hospital. Your vital signs—heart rate, blood pressure, temperature, respiration, and oxygen saturation of your blood—will be constantly monitored. Postoperative care is also similar. You will be removed to a closely supervised recovery room where you are allowed to recover at your own speed from the effects of the sedation and anesthesia. For ambulatory surgery, three to four hours is the norm for sedatives to wear off. You should not expect to drive yourself home after surgery, however. Plan ahead for a responsible adult, perhaps a relative or friend, to pick you up.

THE ANESTHESIA

Whether a local or general anesthetic is appropriate depends on several things: the type of surgery, your preference, and the doctor's judgment. You and your surgeon should be in agreement about the type to be used.

Whatever the decision, you should ask who will administer the anesthesia. It should be given only by an anesthesiologist, a medical doctor trained and certified in anesthesia, or a certified registered nurse anesthetist.

For most cosmetic surgery a local anesthetic is used, combined with an intravenous sedative, or intramuscular sedation. This consists of medication that is injected to induce a relaxed state of well-being and detachment that has best been described as twilight sleep An intravenous apparatus is routinely set up during surgery in case additional sedation is desired. The plastic bottle of clear fluid suspended above the patient contains a saline (salt water) or glucose (sugar) solution that permits the vein to remain open, allowing additional sedation to be given slowly and painlessly as needed without the need for further needle injections. There is no tube (endotracheal) to the lungs, which means you breathe on your own during any routine procedure.

With this type of anesthesia, you may be awake and even aware of what is happening, yet you will feel completely relaxed and at ease. Many of my patients feel such a sense of well-being that they sleep through the entire procedure.

Local anesthesia, particularly on facial procedures, means less chance of developing postoperative complications such as hematoma (a collection of blood under the skin). And usually there is less retching and vomiting later, an important factor for someone who has just had surgery.

It is not unusual, however, for a patient to ask to be "put under" with a general anesthesia. If this is your preference, it is something you should discuss up front with your doctor.

You do not have to make final decisions on the spot. Many patients go home to think over whether they want to go through with the surgery, and many return for more consultations even after they have determined to proceed. You should be sure that additional consultations are included in the cost of the initial fee.

REVIEWING THE BASIC QUESTIONS

Here is a review of the basic questions you should have answered from your initial interview:

- What are the realistic changes you can expect from surgery?
- What are the exact surgical procedures that will take place?
- Will you have ambulatory surgery in the doctor's office and go home the same day or is hospitalization required?
- How long will the surgery take?
- What type of anesthesia will be used?
- Who will administer the anesthesia?
- What are the preoperative and postoperative procedures?
- How long is the period of recuperation?
- What are the medical risks?
- What scarring can you expect?
- What is the cost?

Some other questions I hear frequently are these:

- Is the surgery painful?
- When can I go back to work?
- Will my sex life suffer?
- How soon will I be able to drive?
- When can I wear makeup, wash my hair, bathe?
- Will my face be more sensitive to the sun?
- Will people be able to see that I've had plastic surgery done?
- Will the operation have to be repeated?

All of these are legitimate queries and you should not be embarrassed to ask them or about any small issue that concerns you. No surgery is minor when you are the patient. Of course, the answers to your questions will vary depending on the type of surgery planned. So let's look at the facts about specific types of cosmetic surgery.

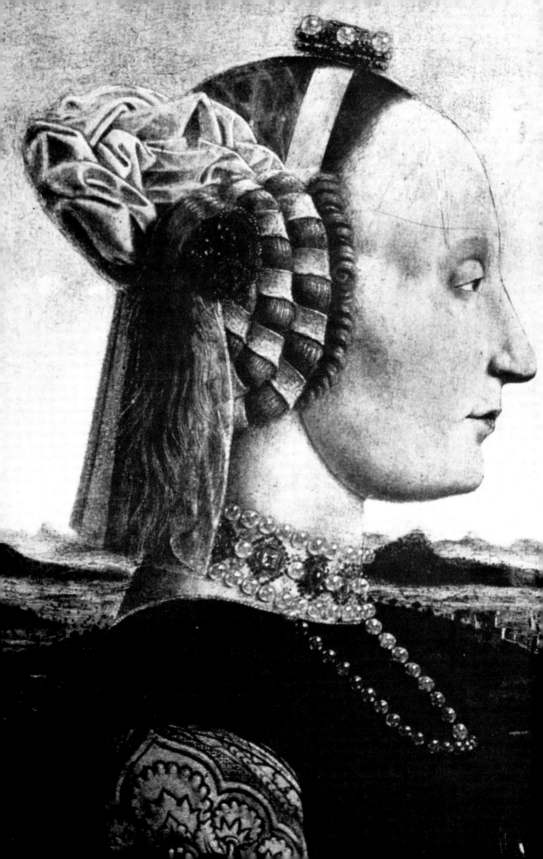

REFINING THE FACE

PART ONE

OVERVIEW OF FACIAL SURGERY 1

*A blemish in the soul cannot be
corrected in the face;
But a blemish in the face,
if corrected,
Can refresh the soul.*

JEAN COCTEAU

The human fascination with faces is as old as mankind itself.

"The love of life is next to the love of our own faces," wrote Sushruta, a Hindu surgeon and teacher, some time before the year 600 B.C.

When Christopher Marlowe was seeking an image to convey the influence of feminine beauty on the course of history, he chose the face of Helen of Troy for one of literature's most famous metaphors: "Was this the face that launched a thousand ships/And burnt the topless towers of Ilium?"

The individuality of every face only deepens our wonder for the complex system of nerves, bone, blood supply, and muscle that makes up the most expressive and communicative part of the human anatomy. Pliny the Elder, the Roman scholar, observed with admiration, "The human features and countenance are so fashioned that there are no two in existence which cannot be distinguished from one another."

From earliest times, we have attempted to read a person's character in the uniqueness of the face. One wonders what modern universities might be like if faculties and admissions officers employed criteria like those of Pythagoras or Socrates in ancient Greece, both of whom accepted students only on the basis of a study of their faces.

Centuries later, English essayist Joseph Addison continued to note, "We may be better known by our looks than by our words . . . a man's speech is more easily disguised than his countenance." He then expressed what ancient philosophers and modern personnel managers have observed in common, "A good face is a letter of recommendation."

The look of the face, then, is something that undeniably affects both our personal and business lives. Tolstoy wrote, "I am convinced that nothing has so marked an influence on the direction of a man's mind as his appearance, and not his appearance in itself so much as his conviction that it is attractive or unattractive."

As a cosmetic surgeon, it is these inner convictions that concern me as much as the outer image, the sense of the self that will inevitably be read in your face by those you encounter. The first work ever printed on the subject of plastic surgery, *De Chirurgia Curtorum* by Gaspare Tagliacozzi (1597), contained a credo that still inspires cosmetic surgeons today, "We restore, repair, and make whole those parts of the face which nature has given but which fortune has taken away, not so much that they may delight the eye, but that they may buoy up the spirit and help the mind . . ."

While cosmetic surgery is as acceptable today as using makeup or hair color, I still meet women who feel guilty about contemplating surgery to improve their appearance, afraid their desire may be seen as empty vanity. Yet wanting to look as good as you possibly can as long as you can is not vanity—it is a sign of healthy self-pride, a normal desire to put your "best face forward." The value is as much inner as outer, for knowing you look your best allows you to face the world with added confidence.

However, facial surgery should not be chosen lightly. Like any surgery, it calls for a thorough understanding of the procedures and a realistic evaluation of the improvements you can and cannot expect.

Facial surgery falls into two categories. Sometimes it is used to correct an imbalance—a nose that is out of proportion to the rest of the face or ears that do not lie flat against the head. Today more people than ever are undertaking surgery such as face-lifts and eyelid surgery not to change their features but to counteract the inevitable changes that come with aging. Many new treatments for the skin are also doing wonders to counteract the unwelcome changes aging brings to the face.

Each kind of surgery will be discussed in the chapters that follow. Read them carefully to gain new insight into the right and wrong reasons for considering facial surgery.

THE FACE-LIFT 2

'Tis a maxim with me to be
as young as long as I can.

The Complete Letters of
LADY MARY WORTLEY MONTAGU

N o one is immune to the effects of aging on the human face.

The process begins gently, almost imperceptibly, as early as age twenty-five or thirty, caused by two of the very forces of nature that keep us on this globe—the force of gravity and the sun. As time robs the skin of its youthful elasticity (with the sun hastening the process), the elastic fibers begin to break and the force of gravity, pulling downward, causes the skin to sag. The more years pass, the more pronounced the sag. In effect, the skin stretches to become too big for the frame it covers, and wrinkles, bags, and jowls are the result.

No cream or potion known to man can return the skin to its youthful trim contours. Only the skill of the cosmetic surgeon can make it fit its frame snugly once again. That is basically what a face-lift accomplishes.

Though aging occurs gradually over many years, changes in the female accelerate quite rapidly with the onset of menopause so that for many women dramatic alterations seem to come almost overnight. When I ask my patients to tell me, in their own words, why they think they need cosmetic surgery, I frequently hear comments like these: "It just happened overnight. Six months ago I didn't look like this." "I woke up one morning and it seemed as though my face fell apart." "I have jowls, bags under my eyes, wrinkles everywhere. Can you help me?"

Most face-lift surgery is performed on patients in their early fifties, but I often see women in their forties who don't like what they see when they look into their mirrors. The average face-lift patient is concerned about the signs of aging in her face, eyelids, jawline, and neck. Ordinarily, she will have the entire face-lift done, taking in all these areas, including the eyelids, although eyes may be done separately and that operation will be treated on its own in the next chapter.

One of the most common complaints I hear involves jowls, overhanging pieces of skin along the jawline that give the face a squarish look. Jowls tend to make male and female faces take on the same shape, as the oval or pear-shaped face of youth disappear, leaving the unisex square face of middle and old age.

Wrinkling in the delicate skin of the neck is one of the most noticeable early signs of aging, as is the "turkey neck," an unattractive condition in which cords of loose flesh become noticeable as bands of skin extending from the lower jaw down to the collarbone.

Some older women also begin to see a hollowness involving their faces, just beneath the cheekbone. This is due to a thinning process in which the deepest layer of the skin, the subcutaneous fat of the face beneath the cheekbone, loses substance, and this combined with the outer skin sagging results in an indentation of the face.

If you are unhappy with the image in your own mirror and think you may be a candidate for face-lift surgery, let's go through some of the basic information you need to know.

THE TECHNIQUES OF THE FACE-LIFT

In face-lift surgery, the skin of the face and neck is freed from the underlying muscle tissue and gently pulled up and back, then narrow strips of excess skin are trimmed, producing a firming of the contours of the face, jaw, and neck when the operation is completed.

The entire procedure, including eyelids, takes about three hours. Many women come to the surgical suite or hospital early in the morning, have their surgery done, recuperate from the effects of the anesthesia, and go home to familiar surroundings the same day, while others prefer to remain overnight in the hospital.

The cost of a face-lift can be anywhere from four to nine thousand dollars, depending on medical costs in the area where you live, the extent of the surgery being done, the age and health of the patient, and other variables.

To prepare the patient for surgery, first the hair is shampooed and the scalp, face, and neck are thoroughly washed with an antiseptic solution of Betadine or Phisohex. Then the face is draped with sterile material. One side of the face is done at a time. The hair is parted by means of a clamp and pushed aside so that the incision can be placed as inconspicuously as possible behind the hairline in the region of the forehead. It is extended down into the crease in front of the ear also, so that the fine scar lines will be hidden in the natural expression lines where the ear and facial skin meet. The line of incision continues around the lobe of the ear, behind the ear, and back into and along the hairline.

The skin of the scalp area is pulled moderately tight by the surgeon, since the hair will conceal these scars. The skin in front of the ear, however, is closed carefully without any tension to avoid distorting the position of the ear and minimize scarring. In both areas the excess skin is removed and the wounds are closed with the fine delicate technique of the plastic surgeon, using fine suture material. The amount of skin removed is very small, but determining the exact amount that will achieve maximum benefit without creating an artificial look is one of the critical artistic judgments that calls for a skilled cosmetic surgeon.

The patient has been given an injection of sedatives that produces the sense of easy relaxation that is called twilight sleep. A local anesthetic is used for the area to be worked on, usually a combination of lidocaine to deaden feeling and epinephrine which controls the amount of bleeding. The face is an area that nature has blessed with a rich supply of blood, and drugs like epinephrine help make facial surgery safer.

Refined techniques have also improved surgery to make the scars less visible. Scarring itself is minimal and the fine scars that are inevitable are easily camouflaged by natural body contours, facial lines of expression, the hair, and the ears.

An additional technique is used when the neck cords have become excessively prominent. It is known as the *SMAS-platysma* procedure because it is the sagging of the platysma muscle in the neck that causes the cords to protrude. This may involve an additional incision under the chin so that the muscle can be tightened or the cords tied together at midline. The actual technique varies according to the specific needs of each patient, but the overall result is to return the muscle to a more normal position.

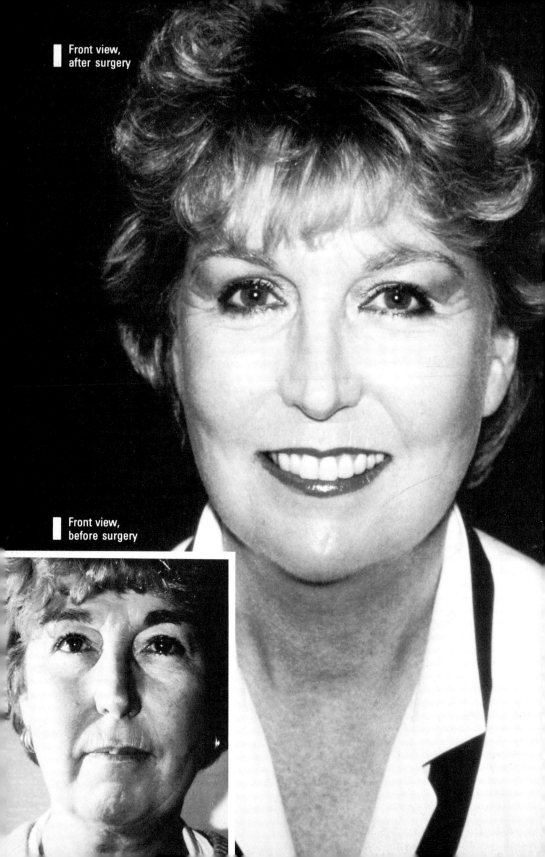

Front view,
after surgery

Front view,
before surgery

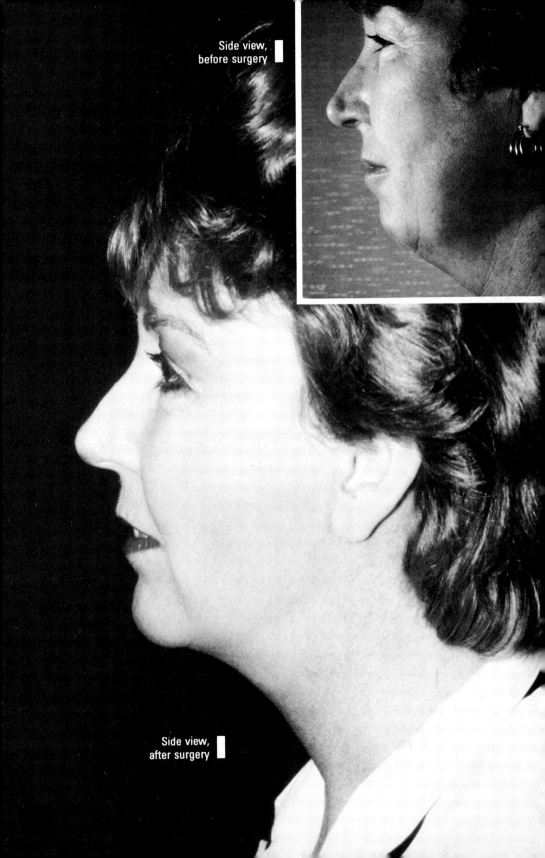

Side view,
before surgery ▮

Side view,
after surgery ▮

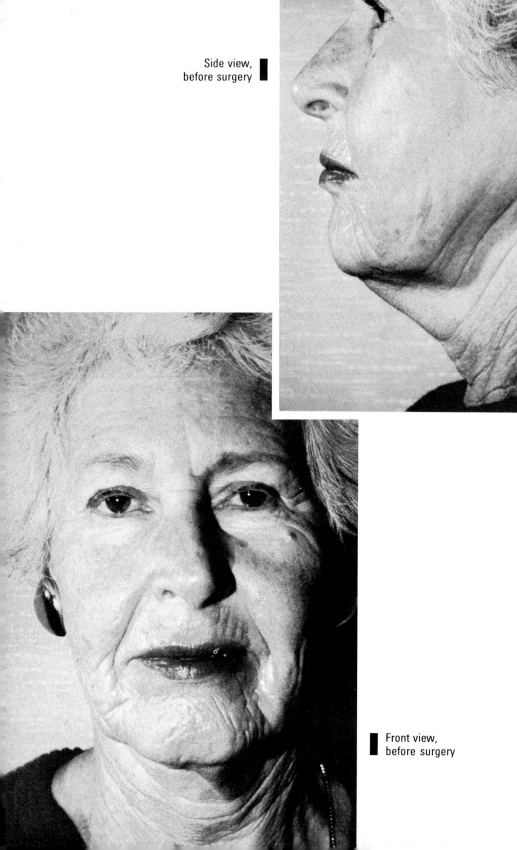

Side view,
before surgery

Front view,
before surgery

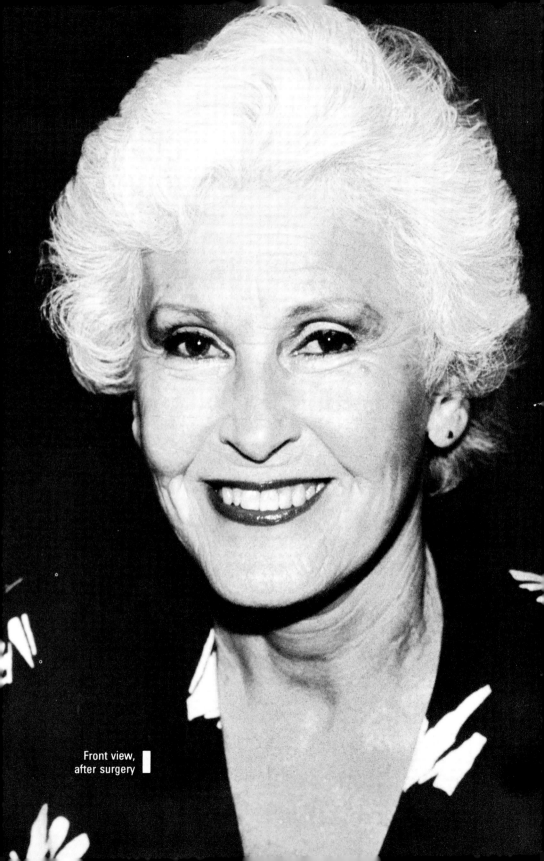

Front view,
after surgery

POSTOPERATIVE CARE

When the surgery is completed, the facial and scalp suture lines will be dressed with a dry sterile gauze bandage. The eyes are not bandaged, but a bland ophthalmic ointment is applied in the eyes to protect them from irritation.

After the operation is completed, the patient is transferred from the operating room to the recovery room, where, under close supervision, she is allowed to gradually awaken from her pleasant twilight sleep. It usually takes three to four hours for the effect of the sedation to wear off. Later that same day, a relative or friend can take the patient home to the comfort of familiar surroundings unless she has chosen to remain overnight in a hospital.

The dressings are removed by the doctor within twenty-four hours. If everything is normal, as expected, an appointment is made within one week for the start of removal of the stitches. The sutures in front of the ear are cut during the first week, the scalp stitches within two weeks.

Following surgery, most patients experience some feeling of tightness and discomfort though there is rarely severe pain. The face is black and blue, and many feel a temporary emotional letdown when they first look in the mirror. As the face heals, these feelings usually are forgotten, but it is important to be aware of what to expect so that you are not alarmed at this normal reaction. The "downer" that often follows surgery is an important reason why I discourage recent widows or divorcées who hope that a face-lift will also lift their grief. I always advise these women to allow time to get themselves back on their feet before undertaking surgery.

There are two big "THOU SHALT NOTS" following a face-lift: NO ICE, ICE PACK, OR ICE CUBE PREPARATION IS EVER, EVER TO BE APPLIED TO THE FACE-LIFT. By using ice or even very cold water, the blood supply to the face can be compromised, causing the facial skin to heal poorly. NO CIGARETTE SMOKING. Smoking also restricts the blood supply to the skin and increases to a great extent the possibility of postoperative complications.

POSSIBLE COMPLICATIONS

Most often face-lift surgery goes quite smoothly. But because the human being is a complicated organism and not a computer that can be programmed, occasionally complications do occur.

The medical condition that is watched for most carefully in any surgery is hematoma or excessive bleeding into the site of the operation. Massive bleeding is rare in a face-lift, however, since no major blood vessel is involved. If bleeding should occur, the surgeon will quickly reopen the suture lines, evacuate the blood clots, control the bleeding, and re-close the wounds.

Other problems that might occur are uncommon and frequently improve over a period of months. These include hair loss around an incision, heavy scarring, and paralysis of part of the face. Since incisions for a face-lift are close to the branches of the nerve that controls the muscles of facial expression, the surgeon must take great care to avoid injuring these nerves, causing paralysis. This possibility, though unlikely, is another reason for great care in choosing a cosmetic surgeon.

Skin slough, an even more unusual complication, happens when there is interference with the blood supply to the operated part of the body. An unsightly scar frequently results that may require surgical correction. Cigarette smoking, which hampers blood circulation, increases the possibility of this occurring. A wound infection requiring drainage and antibiotics may also result.

These are the basic things you need to know about the face-lift. Some of the other common questions I hear from patients concerning postsurgical care are these:

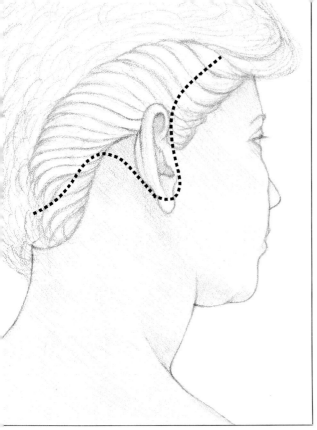

Incisions are made on both sides of the face inside the hairline in the front of the ear around the earlobe and back into the lower scalp.

The skin is pulled up and into the hairline both in front and behind the ear; the excess is removed. In some cases, accumulations of fat are removed from beneath the chin and neck.

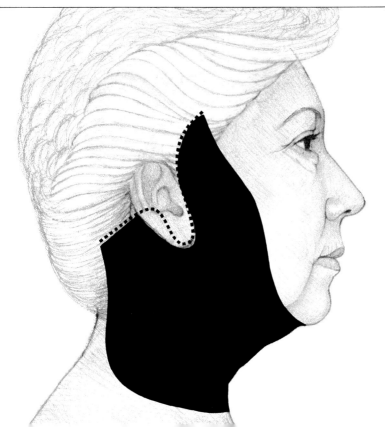

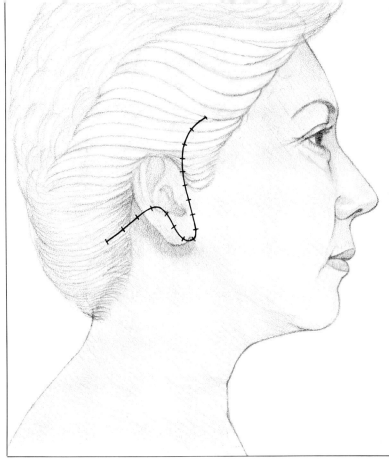

Sutures close the incisions along natural skin lines and creases. Some scars are inevitable, but most will fade and become barely visible.

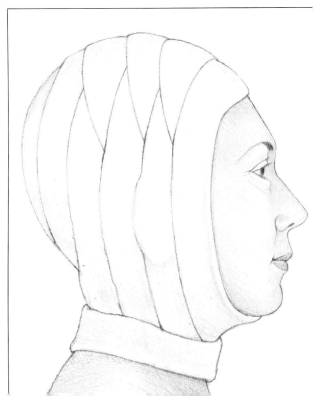

Compressive bandages applied following surgery can be removed within twenty-four hours.

May I wash my hair?

As a woman cosmetic surgeon, I am sensitive to how much better a woman feels when she is able to wash her hair and clean out all the antiseptic and blood resulting from the surgery. I allow my face-lift patients to wash their hair forty-eight hours after surgery. Some physicians prefer a longer wait, some as much as two weeks. However, within six hours surgical wounds usually are sealed (not healed). Unless you are rough or careless or do something to break that fine seal by hard rubbing, washing is perfectly safe and no damage will be done to your new face.

It is important to use a mild soap and to keep the head held back, either in the shower or at the sink as in a beauty salon shampoo, as a precaution to keep the blood from rushing suddenly to the face. The head can be shampooed as often as you like, with careful, very gentle massage of the scalp.

May I dye my hair?

If you regularly bleach your hair, you should do so within a week before surgery. At least a month should pass after surgery before another application. It is best to check this timetable with your own surgeon since individual healing time varies.

When can I wear makeup again?

Since the incisions seal quickly, but are not completely healed for three to six weeks, you can use light makeup the day following surgery by taking care to apply it gently with a brush or sponge only, never with a stick. Heavy foundations are to be avoided and no cream should be massaged into the lines of incision. With prudent and gentle application, however, cosmetics can be used to help conceal bruising and discoloration even during the early healing period.

When will I be socially presentable?

During the first three weeks after surgery you will not be your most beautiful self. There will be varying amounts of black and blue and swelling. Some women are self-conscious about this and feel more comfortable staying out of the public eye. Many women do go out before three weeks have elapsed by wearing makeup, turtleneck sweaters, scarves or wigs, and tinted glasses. An observant eye will still be able to detect that you have had something done to your face but careful camouflage can go a long way.

After three weeks, however, you may be surprised to find that although people will realize you somehow look different, they may not be able to pinpoint the change. They will only know that you look better. Many patients are amused and pleased to hear friends make comments such as "Were you away on vacation? You look rested" or "Did you change your hair style?"

One of my patients who had worried for years about jowls under her chin was amazed that while her friends recognized that she seemed to look younger, they could not immediately see why. "But I was thrilled when I looked in the mirror," she reports. "I knew why."

It will be six months to a year before you see the final, best results from your surgery. The result will be worth waiting for.

When can I drive?

The postsurgery dressing, while it does not immobilize, is a deterrent to the head mobility and vision needed for driving. Once the dressing is removed and stitches are taken out, restoring normal mobility to your head and neck, you can resume driving. Remember that in addition to dressings and sutures, immediately after the operation you will also have a bland ointment in your eyes. Someone else will have to drive you home from surgery.

How long will my face-lift last?

Most face-lifts last an average of seven years, but individual cases may last as few as five or as many as ten years. The face-lift may be repeated any number of times.

When can I exercise?

As with most surgery, strenuous activity is to be avoided for three to six weeks after a face-lift. This means any activity that raises the blood pressure, including sexual intercourse, bending, or lifting. Rely on the judgment of your surgeon for an exact timetable, since some people need less healing time, some more, before they are ready to resume normal activities.

The face-lift will not restore lost youth, but it does remove some of the unwanted "excess baggage" aging brings to the face, leaving a far more relaxed, refreshed, and youthful look. It gives you the confidence that you look your very best—and for most women, that is more than enough reason to consider this procedure.

THE EYELIDS 3

For where is any author in the world
Teaches such beauty as a woman's eye?
From women's eyes this doctrine I derive:
They sparkle still the right Promethean fire;
They are the books, the arts, the academes,
That show, contain, and nourish all the world.

SHAKESPEARE, *Love's Labour's Lost*

I
t has often been said that beauty is in the eye of the beholder, but history and literature tell us that beauty often
is the eye itself. The eyes are the most noticed single feature of the face.

Anthropologists, artists, and writers have all agreed
that the eyes are the most universally expressive facial feature
for the male or female. Even in ancient civilizations, more attention was paid to the eye than to any other single part of the
anatomy. It was considered the center of light, intelligence,
and influence, for good or for evil. The more eyes a deity or
demon possessed, the more power it was considered to wield
over the fate of humans.

The ancient Egyptians credited the eye with complex
powers, as both the symbol of power itself and of the perfec-
tion of the sun. Some Mediterranean fishermen still share the
old Egyptian custom of painting artificial eyes on either side of

the prow of a boat to ward off spirits and to outstare the "evil eye." The Greeks also credited the eye with supernatural qualities of vision and power.

The writings of the New Testament spoke of the effects of the eyes on the physical and spiritual health of the body: "The light (or lamp) of the body is the eye," Mark 6:22. "If thy eye is sound, thy whole body will be full of light," Luke 11:34.

Later poets and lyricists have focused on the eyes as a means of reading the human soul and as reflecting the gamut of emotions from "the look of love" to "green-eyed" jealousy.

Given the fascination with the eyes, it seems only natural that women in all ages of history have tried to enhance the natural attractiveness of their eyes. Once the eyes themselves were dilated artificially with belladonna, a drug no longer used since it has been shown to be potentially harmful to the eye. Ancient Egyptian records reveal what were probably the earliest known experiments in eye makeup. Cleopatra was known to have colored her upper eyelids blue and the lower lids green, not unlike beauties of today, and a black substance called kohl (actually finely powdered antimony sulfide) was used to shape and outline the eyelids and to accent the eyebrows. Even King Tut had a weakness for kohl. When his tomb was opened in the 1920s, a tube of kohl used for eyeshadow was found among the treasures.

It remained for medical research to reveal that, despite all the time and money devoted to eye-enhancing cosmetics from early times to our own, eye beauty sometimes is more than skin deep. There are fat deposits located beneath the skin of the eyelids that defy any concealing with cosmetics. These very real deformities manifested as baggy eyelids or pouches below the lower eye detract from the beauty of the eyes. Surgery is the only procedure to correct this problem.

The first use of surgery to correct eye deformities has been traced to the tenth and eleventh centuries, when Avicenna, a court physician and prime minister to caliphs in Arabia, used primitive techniques to excise from the upper eyelid excess skin that was impairing vision. Early doctors mistakenly believed that this excess fullness of the eyelids was caused by cysts or by an edema, an abnormal accumulation of fluid. Later scientists discovered that it was actually a combination of fatty deposits and drooping skin that usually caused the unattractive pouching. In the early nineteenth century, *blepharoplasty*, or aesthetic upper eyelid surgery (from the Greek word *blepharos* or eyelid), became an accepted fact, setting the stage for the cosmetic surgery to follow.

Though for many the appearance of "bags" is part of the aging process and the relentless pull of gravity on the face, in our own century it was recognized that baggy eyelids or pouches below the eye can be inherited features, not necessarily a result of age.

This condition was partially treated by surgery that became popular from the early 1900s through the flapper generation of the twenties, a procedure sometimes called the miniface-lift. It involved a temporal (at the temples) and preauricular (front of the ears) lift and excision to tighten skin, primarily to correct the small wrinkles of skin at the outside corner of the eye, the familiar and dreaded "crow's feet." From the 1940s the techniques of blepharoplasty have been continually improved and refined to give far better results to the eyelid areas.

Today, many people age forty or older have their eyelids corrected at the same time they have a face-lift. But even earlier, there can be breakdown in the elasticity of the delicate tissues around the eye that would normally keep the fat well beneath the surface of the skin. As a result, a growing number of people in their mid- to late thirties are electing to have eyelid surgery performed alone, long before there is any need for an entire face-lift. They simply want to eliminate the excess skin folds in the upper eyelids and bags beneath the eyes, which detract from the appearance.

Those who have inherited these problems may consider surgery even in their teens. I recently operated on a woman in her early thirties who had the classic "eyebag" look, removing the excess fat from her lower eyelids and tightening the skin to improve her appearance. In one of her postoperative visits, she brought along her nine-year-old daughter who already showed the same deformity. By her midteens, this child will be almost a carbon copy of her mother and will be a candidate for surgery.

Young or old, the problem to be corrected is technically the same: baggy eyelids caused by the herniation or protrusion of the *periorbital* (literally, "around the eye socket") fat, in other words, bulging of the skin of the eyelid and the eyelid muscle due to excessive fatty deposits.

Eyelid surgery is one of the most satisfying of facial plastic surgery procedures. Recovery time is short, the results are long lasting, and the improvement can be dramatic. Because of the proximity to the eye, it is also one of the most exacting operations in cosmetic surgery.

Here are the facts you should know if you are considering this procedure.

THE TECHNIQUE OF EYELID SURGERY

Surgery of the eyelids is usually done under local anesthesia with sedation and normally takes from one and a half to two hours. Fees may range from twenty-five hundred to five thousand dollars, depending on where you live and the complexity of the operation.

The patient is given sedation to induce twilight sleep, a pleasant state of drowsiness and relaxation. The facial skin and the eyebrows are prepared by cleansing with a mild antiseptic solution such as Betadine or Phisohex, and the area to be operated on is surrounded with sterile drapes.

The eyes are often notably asymmetrical. The surgeon carefully points this out in preoperative interviews and in the photographs that are taken before the operation, so that the patient will be familiar with her own asymmetries and the expected changes surgery will bring. To be sure that both sides will be as symmetrical as possible after surgery, the areas where the incisions are to be made are indicated on the skin with sterile marking fluid. A special precise measuring instrument called a caliper is used to ensure accurate measurements.

After the incision lines have been outlined with the surgical marker, the area is injected with a local anesthetic. After about seven minutes, time for the anesthetic to take maximum effect, the incisions are then placed in the normal contours and folds of the face—the fold of the upper lid and beneath the lower eyelash margin—with a view to easier healing and minimal scar effects. Evolution has made the eyelid skin the thinnest skin of the body, thin enough to be able to easily blink to protect the eye. Because it is so thin, it heals beautifully and the scarring from eye surgery normally is so minimal that it cannot be noticed in most patients even without makeup.

The lower eyelid is done first. The incision is placed carefully just beneath the eyelash margin or *ciliary margin* and follows the natural curve of the lower eyelid, extending out into one of the natural laugh lines. Care is taken that the tear duct in the lower eyelid is not disturbed. The actual length of the incision varies with the size of each individual eye and the extent of the skin that will be trimmed or excised. Surgeons determine the exact amount to be excised by using averages based on the age of the patient and a personal evaluation of the extent of excess skin present in each case.

Once the incision has been made, it is deepened through the *orbicularis oculi*, the muscle beneath the eye, and a tiny flap of skin muscle is slit and opened like pages of a book, then laid back with delicate instruments so that the fat below can now be seen easily and removed by the surgeon. The muscle in-

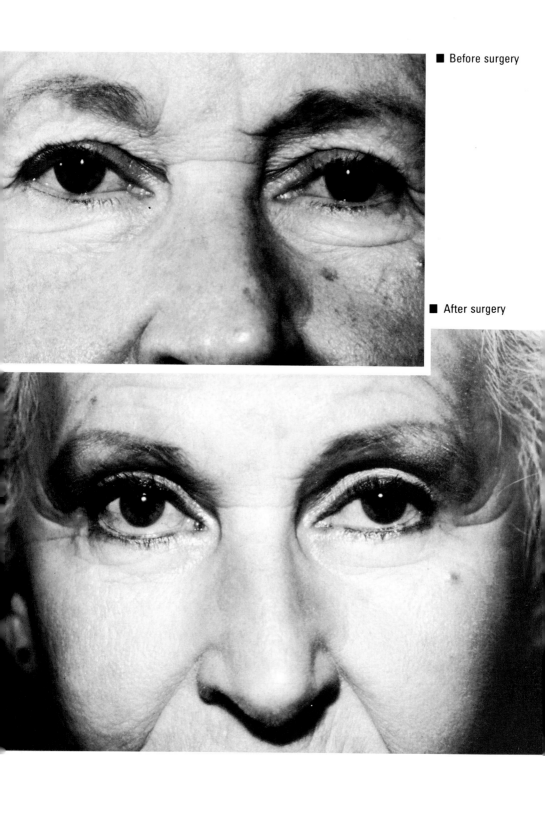

■ Before surgery

■ After surgery

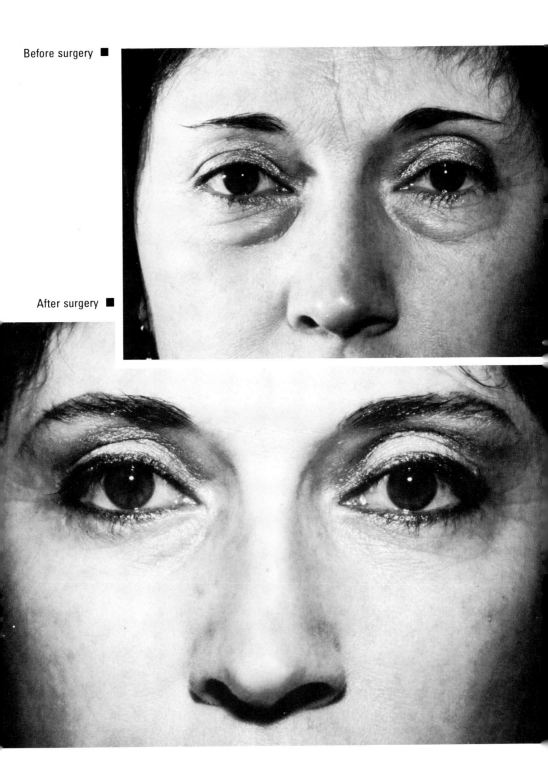

Before surgery ■

After surgery ■

volved is an extraocular muscle that is not necessary to the functioning of the eye.

Three fat pockets are located in the lower eyelid. These are removed in part only so as not to create an unnatural look.

In some patients the muscle underneath the eye is so thick that it produces another large bulky ridge right under the eyelash margin. When this happens, depending on the surgeon's judgment and the patient's perception of the way she would like to look, a portion of this muscle may also be removed. This is often discussed before surgery when the doctor and patient examine her photographs together. This removal causes no interference with eye function.

The incisions are closed with delicate suture material and the surgeon then turns to the upper eyelid. Here the incision is placed in the natural crease so that when the eye is open the fine surgical scar is well camouflaged. There are two pockets of fat in the upper eyelid. These are excised in a manner similar to the technique for the lower lid, again depending on the deformity that is present. The amount trimmed depends on the extent of the patient's deformity.

There may be variations on this technique, depending on the patient's appearance and defects and the surgeon's personal preferences.

Bleeding after surgery is controlled by cauterization with an electric needle, and the wound is closed with fine suture material using the delicate plastic surgery technique.

Different surgeons also use different techniques at the conclusion of eyelid surgery. My own method is to place a bland ophthalmic ointment in the eye in order to protect the globe of the eye. While the eye is still swollen from surgery, it cannot be closed completely and the ointment prevents the globe of the eye from drying out.

There is no bandaging, but gauze sponges moistened with iced saline solution are placed over the operative site to reduce the swelling and the black-and-blue discoloration that is normal after eye surgery. Patients find these cold applications very soothing.

POSTOPERATIVE CARE

Patients are moved into the recovery room after eyelid surgery until the effects of the sedation and anesthesia have worn off. Normally, they are not in a lot of pain, and most of my patients prefer to have this surgery performed on an ambulatory basis, going home the same day in the care of a friend or relative. Many are not even uncomfortable enough to request painkillers, finding that cold compresses are enough to ease their discomfort.

For forty-eight hours after surgery, at regular intervals of about ten minutes every two to three hours, more iced compresses should be applied to the eyelids. I do not like to waken my patients when they go to sleep, but the regular application of these compresses results in a comfortable feeling that is often conducive to better sleep.

After forty-eight hours, warm compresses are applied. The warmth of these must be tested first on the wrist, since the operative site may be numb and could be injured if anything too hot is placed on it.

Care must be taken not to rub the eyes after surgery. Applying compresses usually helps if the eyes feel itchy while they are healing.

Absolutely no medication should be applied in the eye unless the doctor has prescribed it. If an antibiotic ointment is called for, it will be an ophthalmic ointment formulated specifically for use in the eyes. It is important that no ointment be used containing drugs that might cause allergies. The eyes are an integral part of the body and hence can develop an allergic reaction. If a person is allergic to a drug such as penicillin and a penicillin compound is used in the eye, there will be adverse consequences.

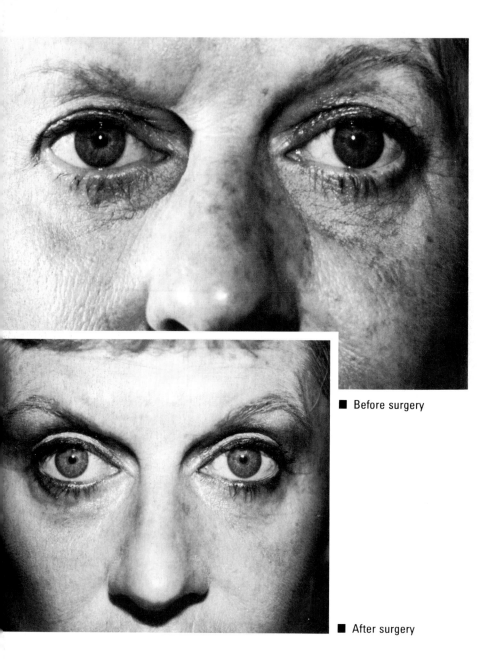

■ Before surgery

■ After surgery

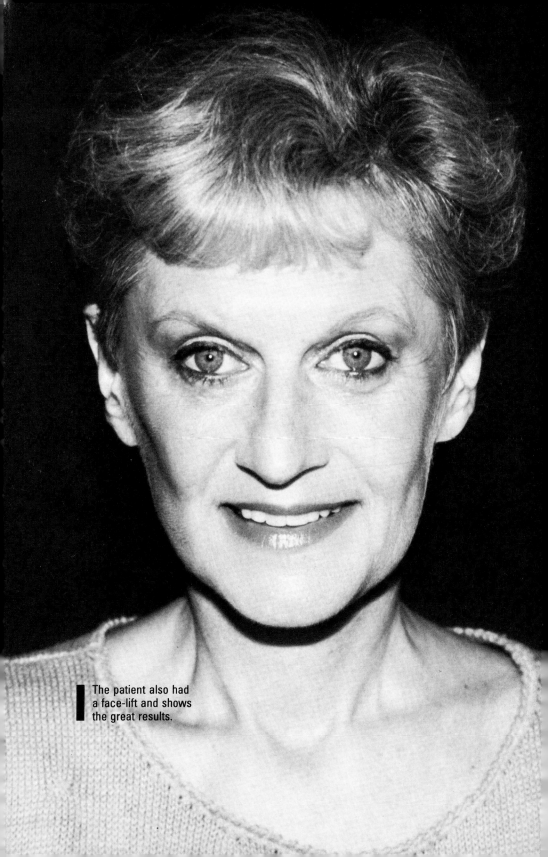

The patient also had
a face-lift and shows
the great results.

All stitches are normally removed within a week of surgery. The patient is advised to relax and take it easy for a few days after surgery and to keep the surgical wound free of soap or shampoo for forty-eight hours. After that, the hair can be washed, so long as the head is not lowered to produce an excessive flow of blood into the operative area.

There will be varying degrees of bruising and swelling for two to three weeks following eyelid surgery. However, many patients do go out, wearing dark glasses to hide their eyes. As with any surgery, strenuous activity is to be avoided for three to six weeks following the operation. This includes any activity that may raise the blood pressure—golf, tennis, or exercise classes, any lifting, pushing or pulling, and sexual intercourse. Those with strenuous jobs should plan to be away or ask for a temporary reassignment for at least three weeks after surgery.

POSSIBLE COMPLICATIONS

Many of the complications that occasionally accompany eyelid surgery are temporary ones, and most can be easily treated. Here are some of the conditions that may arise:

DRY-EYE SYNDROME. Dry eyes, a condition that occurs when there is interference with the production of tears, is an occurrence for many women, even without surgery. Sometimes the eyelid procedure makes the symptoms more bothersome. They are alleviated by using mild eye drops known as artificial tears.

EPIPHORA. The opposite of dry eyes, this condition involves the excessive production of tears because of a disturbance in the mechanical outflow system. It usually clears up on its own without treatment within several weeks after surgery.

CORNEAL INJURY. If the globe of the eye is touched inadvertently during surgery, an abrasion or scrape may occur on the cornea. Antibiotic ointments, night bandaging and the application of eye pads to give the eyes extra daytime rest are prescribed to help an abrasion heal faster.

TELANGIECTASIAS. Many women have the small, superficial blood vessels called telangiectasias. These may increase in size or number after surgery. Corrective makeup such as Esteem by Karen Kimbrough can be used to conceal them.

ENOPHTHALMOUS. If too much fat is removed during surgery, the result may be a sunken eye. The only correction for this is a second operation to graft more fat into the area.

HEMATOMA. The collection of blood in the operative site is a possible complication in any surgery, including eyelid surgery. If this occurs and the amount of blood is small, it can be removed through a tiny incision. If a large amount collects, the site must be opened so that the blood can be evacuated.

A certain amount of letdown is to be expected following surgery. With cosmetic surgery, the normal anxiety and apprehension before any operation is suddenly over, and the mirror reveals not the eagerly anticipated beautiful improvements, but a face covered with black-and-blue bruises. Tears are normal, yet many of my patients are upset when they cry following eyelid surgery, fearful they will injure the surgical site. Fortunately, there is nothing to worry about. In fact, tears may be helpful. They are nature's way of providing a gentle natural bathing of the surgical area.

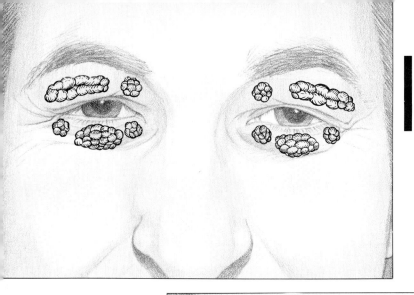

Wrinkled folds of skin hide the upper eyelids, and bags under the eyes are actually deposits of fat.

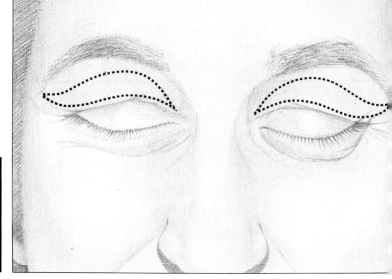

Hairline incisions made in the fold of the upper eyelid and beneath the eyelash margin of the lower eyelid allow for excision of excessive skin and fatty tissue.

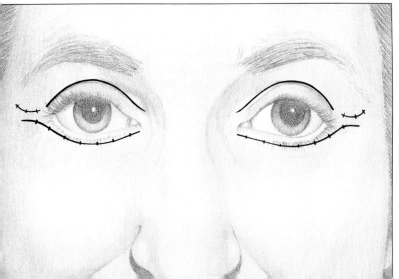

Sutures close the incisions, leaving hairline scars that soon fade.

Before surgery ■

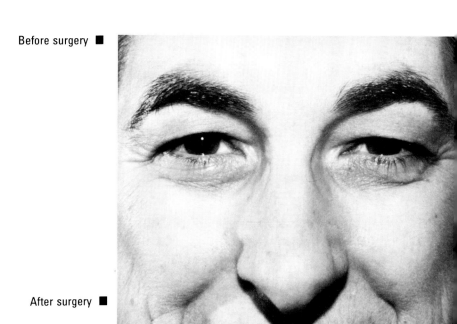

After surgery ■

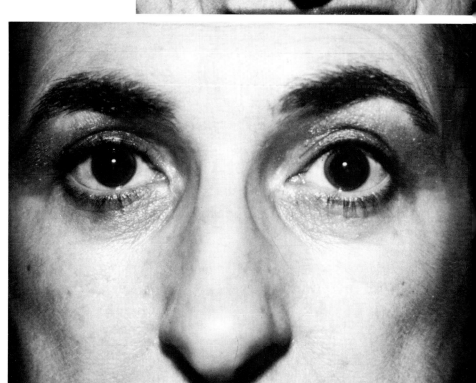

OTHER QUESTIONS ABOUT EYELID SURGERY

Some of the other concerns I hear frequently from my patients are:

When can I wear contact lenses again?

Once the swelling is down and you can manipulate your eye easily once again, it is safe to resume wearing contacts. The healing time varies with the individual, but averages about ten days.

When can I drive?

You can drive when you can see clearly, open and close your eyes normally, and turn your head without any restriction of motion. At a maximum, it takes at least twenty-four hours before tears have washed away the protective eye ointment applied following surgery.

How long will my eyelid operation last?

Unlike face-lifts, which must be repeated periodically, the benefits of eyelid surgery remain for a lifetime. The fat removed does not grow back. Those who have had eyelid surgery and later have a face-lift normally do not have to repeat the eyelid operation unless many years have elapsed since the eyes were done. The only change with time is a certain amount of additional loss of elasticity in the skin that may cause some slight sagging. Occasionally, a patient who has had eyelid surgery early may decide by the time she reaches sixty or sixty-five to have further skin removed, but usually little must be done. I tell my patients that they may want a bit of fine tuning later, but in most instances the eyelid operation does not have to be repeated.

Blepharoplasty, by removing fat pockets and excess skin,

returns eyelids to their normal contours, leaving a woman looking far more relaxed and youthful, with nothing to distract from the beauty of her eyes—yet it can be so subtle a change that no one can pinpoint the reasons for the noticeable improvement.

Far more dramatic are the changes discussed in the next chapter, the recontouring of the nose in the procedure known as *rhinoplasty*.

THE NOSE 4

If the nose of Cleopatra had been a little shorter, the whole face of the world would have been changed.

PASCAL, *Pensées*

hen Samuel Johnson, the English sage, was asked to explain the difference between intuition and sagacity, he replied without hesitation: intuition was the "eye of the mind," whereas sagacity, or shrewdness, was the "nose of the mind."

In our lore, the nose symbolizes being able to "sniff out" the truth, to get beyond the appearance of things to their hidden natures. To have a "nose for news" is high praise for an investigative reporter and to be as "plain as the nose on one's face" is to be very obvious, indeed.

But New England sage Thomas Fuller was recognizing another very important psychological fact when he coined the adage, "He that has a great nose thinks everyone is speaking of it." For while the nose may be less expressive than the eyes and mentioned less in poetic metaphors, it is a crucial and highly prominent feature, one that precedes us wherever we go, an inch or so in advance of the rest of the face.

The shape of the nose does much to determine the overall impression of the face. In his autobiography Charles Darwin writes that he was almost rejected for the voyage of the HMS *Beagle* because the captain did not like his nose, "He doubted whether anyone with my nose could possess sufficient determination for the voyage." And philosopher Arthur Schopenhauer once commented wryly but with some truth that "the fate of so many women depends on a slight up or down curve of their nose." The famous face of Marilyn Monroe might never have made it to the screen had it not been altered by cosmetic surgery when she was twenty-three to take on the perky tilt that was a prerequisite for Hollywood starlets of her day.

The shape of the nose may do much to determine the self-image. Unlike other features, a nose stands on its own. It cannot be hidden or enhanced very well with makeup. When a woman feels that her nose adds to her attractiveness, it buoys her self-confidence, but if she feels her nose is unattractive, that feeling often cannot be allayed by any means short of surgery.

Today, rhinoplasty, cosmetic surgery of the nose, is an accepted fact of life not only for the rich or famous but for many Americans in all walks of life, and the numbers grow each year. More than seventy thousand people had this operation performed in one recent year alone.

Surgery can be performed anytime from about age fifteen, when the nose is completely developed. There is no upper limit, though the older the patient, the longer it takes for the swelling to subside so that the nose can reach its final, best result.

One type of patient I always discourage is a teenager who is being urged into this operation by a parent. I have heard a mother say to an unwilling fifteen-year-old daughter, "You have an ugly nose, and you're going to have surgery before you go to college." This situation is less common than in the past, but I believe it is important that no operation be undertaken until a child is capable of making his or her own decision about whether surgery should be done.

THE IDEAL NOSE

In an initial consultation about the nose two things are to be determined—exactly what you want done and what is both possible and desirable to do from the surgeon's point of view.

Many of my patients come in to see me unsure just what type of new nose they want. They are only sure that they do not like the one they have! It's common to hear simply, "It's too big."

With the help of a mirror and some guidance from the surgeon, the patient can begin to recognize what needs to be done in order to make her more comfortable with the appearance of her nose. I often ask the patient to imagine that she is a sculptor and her nose the clay. I ask her what she would do about changing it. This helps her to visualize and find words and gestures to describe her ideal. At this point, I can give my professional opinion and together we can determine exactly just what is wrong and what can be done to improve it.

As I mentioned earlier, some doctors are using computer imaging to project a new nose contour. I find this is often misleading, because flesh and blood are not the same as an image on a computer screen, and it is often impossible to exactly reproduce a contour from the screen to the face.

Some patients arrive at the doctor's office with something specific in mind, such as taking off a bump, making the nose shorter, or changing a bulbous tip. With these women, I begin by explaining that if you try to change what seems an obvious and isolated defect such as a bump or an elongated tip without altering any of the other substructures that make up the nose, you often end up eliminating one problem only to draw attention to others that are not obvious until after the surgery. When someone has been focusing for years on a noticeable defect, she sometimes does not anticipate that correcting what "sticks out" will only reveal other flaws. In most cases, the best results are obtained when all the substructure itself is changed, at least to some degree. In some cases, nose surgery patients also elect a chin augmentation to further balance the profile, a procedure I will outline in the coming section on surgical techniques.

There are some limitations on what the surgeon can change. Very fine, delicate skin will drape nicely, producing better results than nasal skin that is very thick and oily. The patient needs to be aware of what can and cannot be changed.

Sometimes I see women who request changes that might not improve their appearance in the long run. For example, if a very tall woman tells me she wants a nose that is turned up at the tip, I may advise her against it. She has not realized that because of her above average height, most people she meets would be looking up into her nostrils, which is not an attractive perspective. Even petite women are cautioned today that the little pug nose that was so fashionable twenty years ago is no longer in style.

Standards of beauty do change. The markedly tilted tip and ski slope nose that was the ideal a few decades ago have been replaced with a more or less straight profile. The size of the nose also should conform to the overall size of the person wearing it. Ideally, nose surgery should simply improve and refine the patient's own nose. It should not be a carbon copy shape that was obviously created by a cosmetic surgeon or a rubber stamp of the work of a particular doctor. No one wants to be marked as having had a "nose job."

I spend a great deal of time talking with patients about the appearance of the nose, setting realistic and mutually agreed upon goals for surgery. Taking photographs is particularly helpful in this type of surgery in helping the patient see clearly what should be changed on her own face. Showing catalogs of other people's "before and after" pictures serves little purpose, however, because no two faces or bone structures are alike.

THE TECHNIQUES OF NOSE SURGERY

Rhinoplasty takes approximately one and a half hours in the operating room, and fees range from twenty-five hundred to five thousand dollars. It is helpful to visualize the way the nose is constructed in order to understand the surgical procedures required. While we speak of the nose as a single unit, it is actually composed of three subunits, each comprising about one-third of the total structure. At the top, lying closest to the face are the nasal bones. In the middle third are the upper lateral cartilages, and in the final third, the nasal tip or lobule, with its two-paired alae (cartilage) and septum, the wall of membrane and cartilage that divides the nose in half so that each of the three units has a right and left side. The cosmetic surgeon takes each of these three sections along with the septum into consideration, changing and molding them in order to arrive at the optimal final result for the patient.

The entire area is cleaned with a mild antiseptic and isolated with drapes of sterile material. An injection of sedation is given to lull the patient into the totally relaxed state of twilight sleep. When the sedation has taken effect, the nose is packed with a medication that numbs the inside, and the outer skin is injected with a local anesthetic.

In the last century, external cuts were made on the nose,

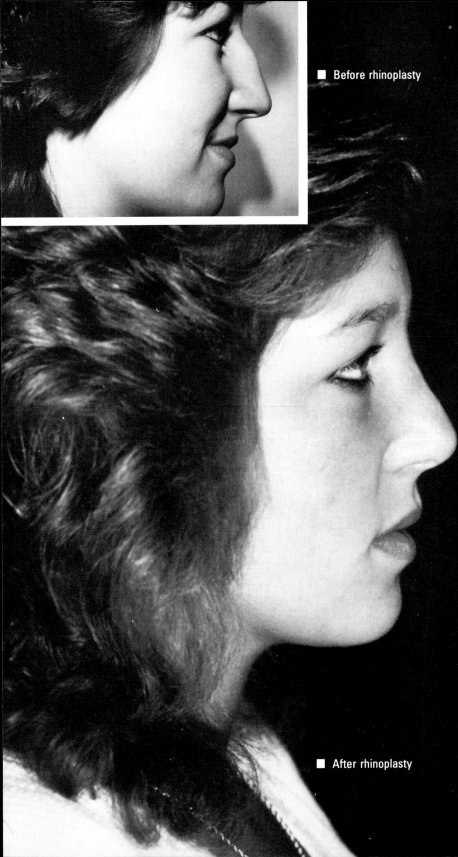

■ Before rhinoplasty

■ After rhinoplasty

leaving telltale scars. Today the incisions are inside the nose, so that normally there is no outer scarring at all. The only exception is when there is too much flare to the nostrils, making it necessary to make an incision in the nasal crease and remove a thin wedge of skin to make the nostrils smaller. This procedure does leave a scar, but since it falls into the crease, it is well camouflaged.

Through the internal incisions, the soft tissues of the nose are separated from the underlying structure of bone and cartilage and this under structure is changed and trimmed to the desired shape.

Care is taken today that excessive cartilage is not removed from the tip of the nose, creating the condition known as a "pinched tip." This was once a common result whose pinched aspect made a subject of cosmetic surgery easy to spot.

Once the dorsal hump, the bone and cartilage that is creating the unattractive profile, is removed, the bones are fractured in order to reconstruct the normal pyramid shape of the nose. This pyramid should occur where the two nasal bones meet. Removing the bump flattens the top of the pyramid and only by breaking and resetting the nasal bones can the correct shape be restored.

The septum of cartilage separating the two sides of the interior nose is rarely straight for its entire length. When there is a significant deviation, enough to crowd the air space and cause difficulty in breathing, it must be straightened surgically in the procedure known as *septoplasty*. This is sometimes done with the rhinoplasty and sometimes later, after the cosmetic changes have healed. Corrective surgery of the septum, when needed to restore proper breathing, is one of the few types of plastic surgery that is often covered by medical insurance plans.

If a chin implant is desired to balance the profile, either a silicone implant or fragments of bone and cartilage from the nose itself can be inserted through an incision in the mouth or through an incision beneath the chin. This often lends more harmony and proportion to the face.

The order of the operative procedure for the nose varies among different surgeons and even one particular surgeon may change his approach depending on the correction that is to be achieved. Even the sequence followed, whether the bump is removed first or the tip is sculpted initially, for example, can produce significantly different results.

POSTOPERATIVE CARE

When the surgery is completed, a packing is placed in the nose and left in place for at least twenty-four hours. A dorsal splint is placed over the nose to reduce swelling and remains usually for one week. The patient is allowed to go home after sufficient time in the recovery room for the effects of anesthesia and sedation to wear off. She is instructed to sleep on the back or side only, with the head slightly elevated.

Because the nasal bones are broken, bleeding into the tissues normally occurs, causing virtually all patients to have black-and-blue eyes after surgery. Only if the tip alone needed correction and no bones are broken can this be avoided. The discoloration requires no special care and will fade naturally in the days following surgery.

Once the splint and bandage is removed, the profile of the nose looks fine, but the face will still be swollen. Patients need to be warned that the swelling that remains on the bridge of the nose creates an optical illusion, making the nose look very wide and the eyes look very far apart. This can be upsetting unless you are prepared for it and realize it is only temporary.

Sometimes nose drops are prescribed to alleviate difficulty

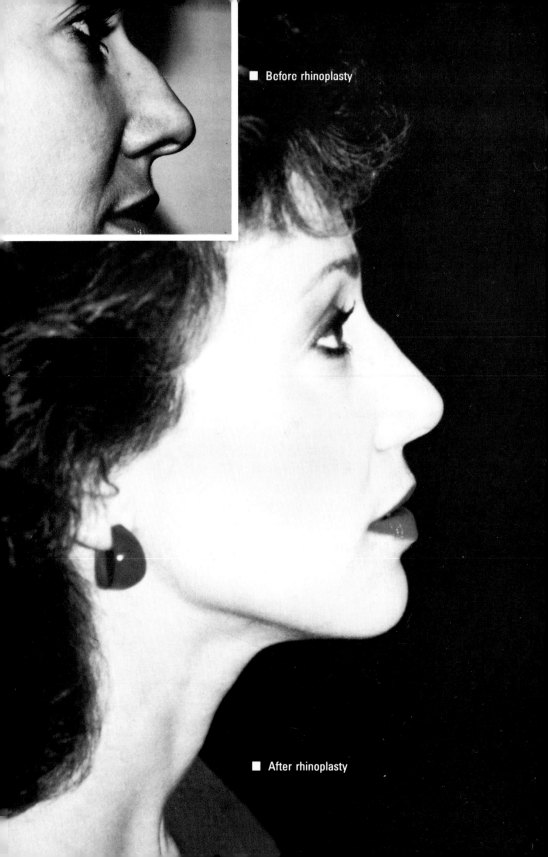

Before rhinoplasty

After rhinoplasty

breathing through the nose, but it is possible to become over-dependent on the relief the drops give from swelling, using drops so often that the mucous membranes inside the nose remain permanently congested. The only way to break this dependence is to go through a withdrawal period when you may not be able to breathe through the nose temporarily.

Only sponge baths are recommended until the dressing is removed, since hot water from shampoos or showers may loosen and dislodge the dressing.

Strenuous activity, including sexual intercourse, is to be avoided for three to six weeks and contact sports should not be played for at least three months after nose surgery. Some patients are comfortable about returning to other usual routines almost immediately, but as with other facial surgery, it usually takes three weeks before noticeable swelling and discoloration disappear. Driving is permitted as soon as the swelling has subsided enough so that the head can be moved freely from side to side and the vision is clear. Obviously, the patient should not expect to drive herself home following surgery.

The skin takes time to shrink and conform to a new underlying bone structure. It will be six months to a year for most patients before the nose is at its final best, and in some cases it can even take eighteen months. This remaining swelling, however, is slight and barely discernible. Most people feel happy and comfortable with their new noses within one month.

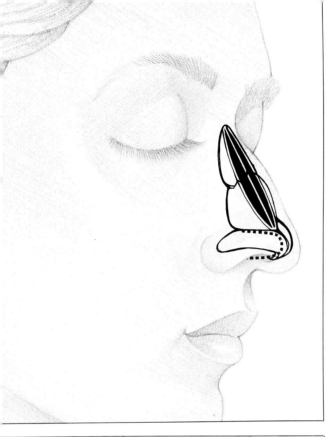

Incisions are made inside each nostril. Cartilage and bone are then cut and reshaped to alter the appearance of the nose.

To reduce the size of the nasal tip, cartilage in the shaded area is partially removed.

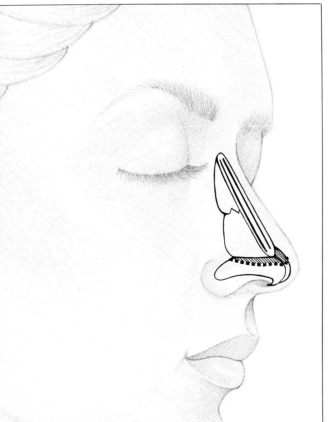

A nasal hump is removed by a saw, chisel, or rasp, leaving the bridge flat, and bones and cartilage spread. Bones are weakened at the base and brought together to form a smooth bridge.

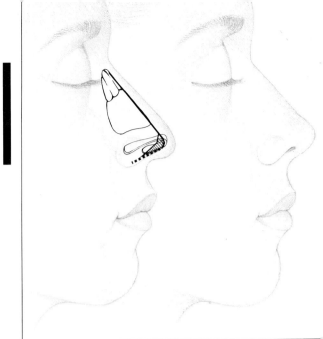

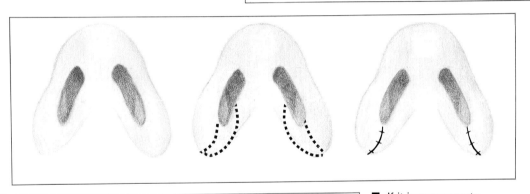

If it is necessary to narrow the base of the nose, wedges of skin are removed and nostrils are brought close to the center. Sutures leave only minute scars.

Application of a splint of tape and plastic or a plaster overlay maintains the new shape of the bone and cartilage.

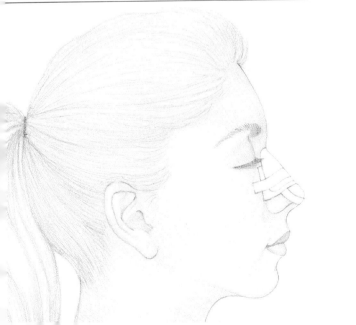

COMPLICATIONS

Nasal bleeding is the most common complication following surgery. But that doesn't mean it happens frequently. Usually it can be handled at home with sedation and iced compresses. If bleeding becomes serious, hospitalization may be necessary.

Occasionally, the whites of the eyes turn red due to blood leaking from the nasal area to the subconjunctival layers of the eye. Other than being unattractive, this discoloration is not harmful and does not interfere with vision. It usually disappears within a month with no after effects.

Small pimples are a minor annoyance that may develop beneath the bandage because the patient has not been able to wash underneath it. Once the bandage is off and the area can be given attention, the skin quickly returns to normal.

Occasionally, circumstances beyond the surgeon's or patient's control may produce minor irregularities such as contour defects or a slight asymmetry of the nose following surgery. These can usually be corrected through minor revisions, though occasionally the entire rhinoplasty must be redone.

The improvements from nose surgery are permanent and the operation does not have to be repeated. Once the nose is broken, however, it is more susceptible to future trauma, so it takes less force to rebreak it. For that reason, young people planning to play football or other contact sports, are advised to wait until their sports careers are over before having their noses done.

The only other surgery that might be elected later would be due to the effects of aging. Like the skin of the face, the skin of the nose loses its elasticity over the years. As a result, the nose appears to be getting longer, and in a sense it is, in fact, lengthening. When this happens to a patient who is planning a face-lift, the surgeon may shorten and elevate the nose slightly at the same time to return a more youthful appearance to the face. Shortening requires only inside incisions so no external mark or scar results.

For most patients, rhinoplasty results in a remarkably happy improvement that achieves exactly what both the patient and the cosmetic surgeon hope for—a woman who feels much better about herself.

THE EARS AND LIPS 5

There was a young man of Devizes,
Whose ears were of different sizes;
    The one that was small
    Was of no use at all,
But the other won several prizes.

LANGFORD REED, *The Limerick Book*

THE EAR No part of the body is a more marvelous blend of form and function than the human ear.

The ear's shell-like construction of whorls and tunnels efficiently captures sound waves and funnels them to the auditory canal. It also protects the inner ear from damage.

These delicate and purposeful shapes have fascinated both musicians and poets. Musical terms such as *tympanum* and *drum* have come to be the common names for parts of the ear's inner structure. Words such as *helix* (the outer border of the ear), *antihelix* (the inside border structure) and *concha* (the opening to the passage to the inner ear) are all poetic words inspired by the ear's striking resemblance to a shell.

The ear's important function in allowing us to communicate with our world through hearing has also been duly noted. Geoffrey Chaucer is credited with two sayings still in use today, "In one ear and out the other," and an early version of the belief the ears "burn" when someone speaks of us in our absence, "We shall speak of thee somewhat, I believe, when thou art gone, to make thine ears glow."

To be "all ears" was said approvingly by the seventeenth-century poet Milton, but Aristotle much earlier revealed a popular negative judgment, that large ears betrayed "a tendency to irrelevant talk or chattering." and in *Twelfth Night*, when Maria says contemptuously to Malvolio, "Go shake your ears," she is comparing him to a foolish ass.

Large or small, the ear is a unique feature. No two people have ears exactly alike and even a person's own two ears are not identical. There are anthropomorphological differences as well. The longest and widest ears are found among Asians, and inhabitants of the far north, including Alaskans, Aleuts, and Eskimos. Blacks' ears are the shortest. Caucasian ears are of medium length but similar to blacks' ears in width. In Japanese people, it is common for the lobule to be attached to the skin of the neck, while Caucasian and black lobules usually hang free.

While the ear has inspired adornment with jewelry and ornaments from the earliest recorded human history, it is normally an inconspicuous feature whose individual differences may go unnoticed on their own, particularly on women whose hair covers the ear. Perhaps that is why when abnormalities do occur, this unobtrusive feature can become a particularly embarrassing focal point.

Among congenital ear defects, *protruding ears* are the most common complaint. Other deformities that sometimes occur include *microtia*, a nondeveloped ear, and *cryptotia* or pocket ear, which occurs when the ear adheres to the skin, holding it too close to the scalp so that the structure of the ear is not clearly defined. *Satyr ears*, like those of Mr. Spock in "Star Trek," are pointed at the tips, *lop ears* droop downward at the top, *Machiavellian ears* occur when the helix and antihelix are not properly formed, and *shell ears* are another malformation involving lack of definition of the ear structure.

The condition known as *cauliflower ears* is the result of trauma to the ear, most commonly caused by automobile accidents, severe falls, or blows from fistfighting, the latter accounting for the large number of boxers who develop this problem. Cauliflower ears occur when injury causes bleeding into the tissues of the ear. The blood forms a hematoma (a collection of blood in a confined space) causing lumpy scar tissue to develop which may deform the ear. Such hematomas are treated as surgical emergencies. If they are not properly drained, cartilage-damaging infection may set in. Once extensive destruction of the cartilage occurs, it is difficult to find enough cartilage available elsewhere on the body to allow for successful reconstructive surgery.

Another acquired deformity is the *bifid* or *cleft lobule of the ear,* caused when an earring in a pierced ear somehow is pulled all the way through the earlobe. The ear will heal, but the lobe will remain split. To correct this condition, the surgeon must first make little flaps, then join the flaps smoothly to avoid notching.

Ears should never be pierced by inexperienced or non-surgical personnel. Cysts may form if the outer skin is forced inside the lobe and soreness, lumps, or infection may follow. Chronic infection is also a possibility if ears are pierced improperly. Multiple ear piercing is a current fad, with people adorning each ear with three, four, or even five earrings. I find this disturbing, because once the fad passes, the scars of the ear will be permanent. It is wise to consult your physician about the right way to have your ears pierced.

CANDIDATES FOR EAR SURGERY

Most of my ear surgery (*otoplasty*) patients are young. The most common reason for this kind of surgery is protruding ears that stick out from the head. This is a defect that is quickly evident and best corrected early whenever possible, before a child enters school and becomes subject to teasing by classmates. Four, an age when the ear is 85 percent developed and is large enough for the surgeon to work on easily, is an ideal time for surgery. At age four or five, the child is usually up and ready to go within a few hours after surgery and heals beautifully and quickly.

However, it is never too late for otoplasty. Many adults have lived with this condition for years, never realizing until middle age that anything could be done to help them. Others had parents who refused to have the surgery performed and had to wait until they were psychologically and financially independent enough to make the decision to have surgery for themselves. At any age, it is an operation with many psychological benefits. Ears that stick out can be the target of much painful ridicule.

TECHNIQUES FOR EAR SURGERY

Otoplasty is performed under local anesthesia with sedation. Fees range from two thousand to forty-five hundred dollars. If the patient is fearful, as young children often are, general anesthesia can be used. The procedure can be performed in a one-day stay in the hospital, but with very strict instructions to the parents to be aware of symptoms that might indicate problems, such as severe pain that could mean bleeding into the operative site, leading to hematoma formation.

Usually both ears are done at the same time even if only one seems to need correction. This is done to assure symmetry. If only one ear is changed, the other often seems out of align-

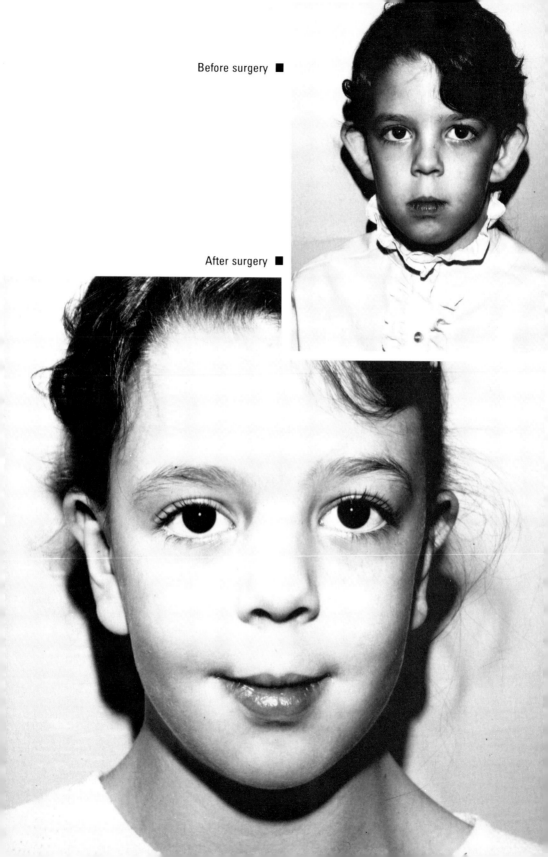

Before surgery ■

After surgery ■

ment afterward, even if it appeared normal before the operation.

Some people think that correcting protruding ears simply means pulling the ear closer to the head and sewing it into place. This actually is the way the operation was first performed in New York in 1881. However, it was not a satisfactory procedure. Ear cartilage has spring, and it eventually pulls on the skin. Since the skin is elastic, it gives in to this pull eventually, allowing the ears to return to their original position.

Skillful otoplasty as it is done today is a truly aesthetic procedure. The ear is not only permanently placed closer to the head, but any structures that are underdeveloped or overdeveloped can be tailored and restructured to form a normal ear shape.

To correct protruding ears, the fibers on the front of the cartilage are divided and weakened, leaving the natural pull of the stronger fibers on the back with more power to bend the ear back naturally toward the head. To weaken the front cartilage, the surgeon cuts it, breaking the natural springiness that has propelled the ear forward.

The incision is usually made behind the ear so that there are no marks or scars that are easily seen. In cases where front incisions are required, they are placed in a fold or natural crease so that the resultant scar simply follows the normal ear crease.

Any cartilage that has not folded properly to create a normal ear contour is also cut so that it can be adjusted. In the case of lop ears, where the antihelix is not unfurled, the surgeon works through the incision behind the ear to recontour the cartilage from the overlying skin, actually molding it to create an antihelix. If some of the cartilage must be removed to create a normal shape, sutures are used to hold the remaining cartilage in place.

Cup ears are usually corrected by removing excess cartilage in the concha. Shell ears are reformed by thinning the cartilage along the back edge of the ear causing the tissue to curl forward. For satyr ears, the pointed section is trimmed or tubed and sutured into shape.

POSTOPERATIVE PROCEDURES

After the operation, the patient is taken to the recovery room and given ample time to recover from the sedatives. No ice or heat is used, just a head dressing that covers the ears and goes around the head like a football helmet. It is very similar to a face-lift dressing. Because the ears are covered, hearing is slightly affected until the dressing is removed.

There are no restrictions on sleeping positions. Pain is not usually excessive, and after twenty-four hours patients seldom need any pain medication.

The helmet dressing comes off in one week; the sutures will be taken out in from one to two weeks, depending on how quickly the wound heals. Once the dressing has been removed, the hair can be washed, using care and gentleness near the operative site. Driving also can be resumed when the dressing is off and the head can be turned comfortably from side to side.

With ear surgery, it does not take weeks or months to see good results. When the ear dressing is removed, the newly sculpted ear is easily visible and seen as corrected. Sometimes the patient is advised to wear a ski band while sleeping for several months following surgery, and there is a certain amount of bruising and discoloration, but it is not usually excessive. By the time the dressings are off and the patient goes out in public, it is not immediately obvious that plastic surgery has been performed.

The improvement is permanent. Even when the operation is done at a very young age, the corrected ear grows normally along with the rest of the child's body.

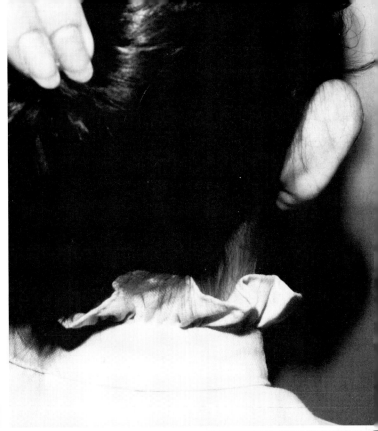

Back view,
before surgery

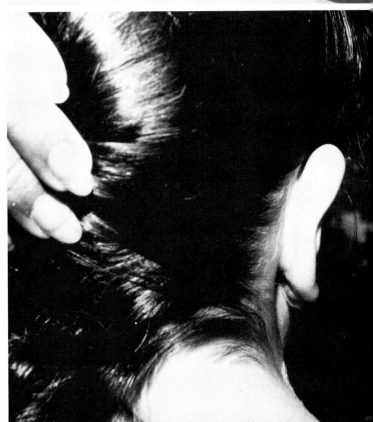

Back view,
after surgery

POSSIBLE COMPLICATIONS

The complication most closely watched for in ear surgery is hematoma or bleeding into the operative site. If this occurs, blood must be drained quickly because of the possible production of a secondary perichondritis, infection of the fibrous connective tissue of the cartilage, which can lead to loss of cartilage tissue. If the bleeding is not checked and excessive scarring occurs, the condition known as cauliflower ear may result, just as it does when bleeding is caused by a blow.

Sometimes a new deformity can result from a corrective operation, if an ear is pulled back too much or too little. Overcorrection produces what is known as the "telephone deformity," which looks as though someone had pressed a telephone receiver too hard against the ear. This is infrequent, but when it does occur, the only remedy is further surgery.

As a rule, however, ear surgery goes smoothly with few complications and highly gratifying results.

THE LIPS

Lip surgery is less common than other types of facial operations, but it is no less important to those who seek it. Lips are highly visible features. Any noticeable abnormality is doubly distressing because the lips are so vitally important to speech. Everyone lip-reads on occasion when trying to understand another person, so a lip impediment limits the ability to communicate clearly.

Most often, cosmetic lip surgery is performed because the patient feels her lips are too large. The cause may be congenital, a racial characteristic, a reaction to illness, or a glandular disorder.

Lips that are too fleshy can be recontoured in a straightforward procedure that is usually done on an ambulatory basis, either in the surgeon's office or as an outpatient in a hospital. The procedure, known as *cheiloplasty*, takes about one and a half hours and the fees for lip surgery range from one to three thousand dollars.

An incision is made on the inside of the lip from one corner of the mouth to the other and soft tissue from the inner lining of the lips, called *mucosa*, is removed. The incision is then closed with sutures. Tissue may also be added for lips that are abnormally thin. Local anesthesia is usually used for these procedures and the bleeding is carefully controlled.

There is often excessive swelling after a lip operation, so a soft diet is an essential part of postoperative care.

Sometimes a lip problem is part of a deformity that also involves the chin, jaw, and teeth. When this is the case, these problems are usually corrected before lip reconstruction is considered.

There is a final category of facial surgery to be discussed in the next chapter that does not involve changing specific features. Instead, it involves the removal of scars or a variety of disfiguring growths and swellings that I've come to label "lumps and bumps."

LUMPS, BUMPS, AND SCARS 6

He jests at scars that never felt a wound.

SHAKESPEARE, *Romeo and Juliet*

LUMPS AND BUMPS *Lumps* and *bumps* are two of the oldest words in the English language. Today, they are often used by cosmetic surgeons to lump together the variety of visible swellings of the skin that may plague us, from the common mole to benign or malignant tumors.

Wen, an old term now referring only to sebaceous cysts, was once used to cover this whole range of visible growths and swellings. In the hands of early writers, it often became the stuff of comedy.

The English scholar Addison reported that Cicero had "a little wen on his nose." Charles Dickens in *The Old Curiosity Shop* describes one of his characters as "a tall meagre man, with a nose like a wen." Shakespeare's Prince Hal refers fondly to the swollen form of his friend Falstaff when he says, "I do allow this wen to be as familiar with me as my dog!"

But while writers may refer to such disfigurements with humor, few people who have them take them lightly. A growth is always cause for concern. When patients ask a plastic surgeon to excise their "lumps" and "bumps," especially from the face or neck, they are concerned with appearance, but even more concerned that the offending lumps may prove to be signs of a serious problem.

Let's take a look at some of the most common causes of swellings on the skin and their treatment.

Nevus refers to a growth or mark on the skin that may be due either to an excess or deficiency of tissue. The variety we are most familiar with is the mole, which is a circular malformation colored by pigment. It is usually dark, slightly raised from the skin, and sometimes hairy. Moles on the body are very common and may be harmless. If they are on the face or neck and are aesthetically displeasing, however, they can be easily removed surgically. Smaller moles also may be burned off with an electric tool or frozen off with dry ice.

While most moles are benign, some can be premalignant or even malignant. Here are some warning signs of changes in a mole that could herald potential trouble, reasons for a speedy examination by a doctor:

- bleeding
- change in color, either lightening or deepening
- change in size
- irregular margins
- ulceration

Any of these symptoms may cause the doctor to recommend that the growth be surgically removed.

Plastic surgeons see a range of the growths known as *cysts*. A cyst is any sac containing a liquid. Among those that most frequently occur are:

Epidermoid cysts are tense smooth swellings containing a

cheesy lipid rich material. The cyst is attached to the skin but fully movable over the underlying tissues. These vary in size and tend to occur on the face, neck, and trunk. They are removed by simple surgical excision.

Sebaceous cysts or wens are raised sacs containing sebum, a fatty lubricant secreted by the sebaceous glands of the skin. They occur frequently around the scalp and neck simply because of the high concentration of glands in these areas. They are also removed surgically.

Milia or whiteheads are tiny, superficial cysts located most frequently around the eyes. They contain *epidermal* or skin material which is simply removed by breaking the skin and scooping out the contents of the cyst.

A *tumor*, by definition, is a new growth of tissue forming an abnormal mass that serves no physiologic function. They develop independent of and unrestrained by the normal laws of growth, and with very few exceptions, their cause is unknown. Tumors may be benign, meaning harmless, or malignant, meaning that they tend to spread or *metastasize*, destroying surrounding or distant tissue.

Benign tumors sometimes may be *fibrous tumors*, seen as small elevations on the skin which can be easily removed. Other common types are *papillomas*, which are attached to the skin by a tiny slender stalk which may be clipped away, and *lipomas*, made up of a collection of fatty cells. Lipomas frequently occur in multiples. If you have one, several more usually follow.

Until recently, the usual treatment for all benign lipomas was surgical excision, but today suction lipolysis may be a simpler way to remove them. A small incision is placed in a body fold or crease near the lipoma and the lipoma is simply siphoned out. Since the incision is smaller, the scarring will be less than from the usual surgical incision. If the growth is located in an area of high visibility, the incision may be done in a body crease distant from the site in order to camouflage the resultant scar.

Malignant skin cancers are a growing medical concern. They are caused primarily by overexposure to the sun and are appearing in epidemic numbers, the price we are paying for our sun-worshipping society.

Basal cell carcinoma, the most frequently seen skin cancer, is a malignant tumor made up of *epithelial* or skin tissue. It is especially common in fair-skinned individuals who have only a small supply of *melanin,* a pigment that protects the skin from damaging sun rays. This is the slowest growing and most contained of the cancerous skin tumors.

Two more serious cancer types are the *squamous cell carcinoma* and the *melanoma,* the most dangerous of all skin cancers. Each of these metastasizes or spreads more rapidly to invade surrounding or underlying structures and even distant body parts.

Both basal and squamous cell carcinomas first appear as ulcers or small sores that fail to heal. Melanomas tend to be blacker in color and irregular in outline. They may be ulcerated or variegated. Often they are seen as moles that are changing in character.

Malignant tumors must be surgically removed, along with a safety margin of surrounding normal tissue to be sure that all cancerous cells are excised. If the lesion is located on a part of the body that allows for easy removal and closure, the procedure is relatively simple. However, when the tumor is located near a vital organ such as the eye, nose, mouth, lips, or ear, the highest skills of the plastic surgeon may be called into play. For example, if a major portion of an eyelid has to be sacrificed to separate healthy tissue from diseased cells, major reconstructive techniques are required.

BIRTHMARKS

Sometimes unwanted growths are with us from birth. Capillary *hemangiomas*, which include "port wine stains," actually are a form of benign tumors. They are flat birthmarks that look like flat wine-colored patches on the skin. These are distressing when they occur on the face, and until recently little could be done about them. However, laser treatments are creating great hope in this area. The treatments are not widely available as yet, so long waiting lists are not uncommon. Ask your physician about the possibility of laser treatment in your own area.

Strawberry *hemangiomas* are similar reddish birthmarks that are raised above the level of the skin rather than flat. They often disappear by themselves by about age five, so parents frequently are advised to wait before they seek treatment for their children. In some instances, however, the hemangiomas grow rapidly instead of disappear. When this occurs near the mouth so that breathing is obstructed, or near the eye so as to block vision, sophisticated surgery is required. If hemangiomas occur in such critical areas, it is best to seek early medical advice before growth occurs. One successful early treatment is with applications of dry ice, which kills the underlying cells, preventing any further growth. Usually, however, even without intervention, the bright color pales, and as the child grows, the raised mark flattens to be hardly noticeable. A recent innovation in the treatment of birthmarks is skin expansion. Normal skin next to the lesion is stretched out over several weeks by instilling salt water into a balloon that has been placed beneath the normal skin. When adequate expansion occurs the defect is removed and the stretched-out skin is then rotated into the area and the final reconstruction performed.

SCARS

Scars are a perfect example of the old adage that beauty is in the eye of the beholder. In some native cultures, scars are considered beautiful and people deliberately scar their bodies as a form of adornment. Scars—often arranged in ornate designs—have been used also to convey tribal messages, to denote caste or rank, and even as charms to ensure a successful love life.

Most modern men and women, however, find nothing attractive about the scars they bear from accidents, illness, or surgery. While all scars are permanent, the plastic surgeon often can offer ways to minimize and camouflage, making the scars much less prominent. This is known as revisional surgery.

Scars fall into two general types. Those caused by accident or illness may occur on any part of the body. Scarring resulting from a severe case of acne is concentrated on the face and chest. Treatments vary, depending on both the cause and location of the scar.

When a scar is raised or jagged, excision and revision may help. This means simply that the scar is cut out and the edges sewn together more skillfully to produce a straighter, smoother result.

Z-Plasty or *W-Plasty* are mainstays of the plastic surgeon's art. They are techniques used to place scars in a normal body crease or facial expression line where they are less likely to be noticed. These same techniques also can be used to change the location of an existing scar, making it less visible.

Larger scars from an appendectomy or cesarean section also can often be moved by the more complex tummy tuck operation (see chapter 11, The Abdomen). While not all scars will disappear, they are relocated below the bikini line, where they seldom show. Gallbladder scars are more difficult to eliminate, but at least they are moved below the naval and made less obvious.

Dermabrasion, in laymen's terms, is sanding. It is sometimes used to treat acne scars and traumatic facial scars. Dermabrasion is done with a cylinder-shaped instrument driven by air. This hand-held instrument has a rough surface which actually rubs down the superficial layers of skin, causing scars to blend in better. It is a technique that should be used only by a skilled professional.

Acne scars are also frequently helped with a face-lift. People who suffered from severe acne in youth frequently show premature aging signs in the face. The reason is that acne scars, which can involve the full thickness of the skin, may lessen the skin's elasticity by actually destroying elastic fibers. Radiation treatments used in the past for severe acne cases may also damage the skin.

Recently I performed a face-lift on a patient who had undergone radiation treatment for acne in her teens and who, although she was around forty, appeared much older. A vast amount of excessive skin had to be removed. The result not only restored a far more youthful appearance but stretched the acne scars, giving the face a much smoother look.

Other small skin depressions, such as scars left by chicken pox, may be filled out with injections of collagen. We will talk in detail about other uses of collagen and dermabrasion in the next chapter on skin care.

Often more than one technique may be used to minimize scarring. For example, many people involved in automobile accidents emerge with multiple, small, superficial cuts from shattered glass and minute fragments of glass actually embedded in their wounds. Sometimes the whole side of the face may be covered with these small, multiple scars. Treatment might consist of excision-revision on the larger scars, followed in about six months by dermabrasion to minimize the remaining marks.

Revisionary surgery is usually done under local anesthesia on an ambulatory basis in a doctor's office or as an outpatient in a hospital. The cost varies considerably, depending on the procedures required.

Like any wound, scars take time to heal fully. Revisional surgery should not be considered until the healing process is complete, normally a period of six months to a year. Over this time, a scar that is red, elevated, and hard to the touch may fade and flatten as the surrounding tissue softens. And it should also be remembered that revisionary surgery will leave its own scars, which must be given time to heal. The best results will not be seen for a period of months after surgery.

Some of the nonsurgical techniques used to diminish scars, such as collagen and dermabrasion, can also be used to ward off unwanted signs of aging. They are part of many exciting developments in skin care that are now available to aid the cosmetic surgeon in helping you look your best. Let's look at some of these new and exciting techniques.

AGING AND THE SKIN 7

Good looks come only with care,
and die if neglected.

OVID

E very woman is born with beautiful skin. As the years pass, however, that baby smooth complexion slowly alters to become the most visible record of the passage of time. Even plastic surgery, while it can correct sagging facial contours, cannot alter the inevitable changes in the texture and tone of the skin.

But there is much that can be done to slow the unwelcome lines and wrinkles, discolorations, and blemishes that come with age. As I have observed the remarkable difference in appearance in women who have taken good care of their complexions, I have become more and more convinced that proper skin care can be the most important single factor in maintaining youthful good looks.

Many people don't recognize the importance of the skin and its many functions in helping us adjust to our environment. This remarkable organ, when laid out flat, would measure some twenty square feet for an average adult. With fifteen feet of blood vessels per square inch, the skin acts as the body's thermostat, regulating its temperature. It is the first line of defense against harmful germs as well as a waterproof sac that prevents the loss of water, blood, and other essential body fluids. It is also an organ of excretion, continually eliminating body wastes through more than 2 million sweat pores.

Proper skin care means simply helping this marvelous organ to do what it does naturally—to renew itself every single day. Though the skin measures less than an eighth of an inch even at the thickest points, such as the soles of the feet, if you could look at your skin through a microscope, you would see that it is made of several distinct layers. An extra layer of fat underneath provides a cushion and gives the skin a springy, youthful texture.

The *dermis*, the deepest layer, is made of tough connective tissues, elastin, and collagen, which account for the elasticity in the skin. This layer also contains the sweat and sebaceous glands. Sebaceous glands produce an oil called sebum, and send it to the surface through the pores, where it combines with the moisture from the sweat glands to produce a mixture called the acid mantle. It is this acid mantle that keeps the skin supple.

The *epidermis*, the layer of skin we see, actually has five sublayers of its own. The minuscule cells that make up the skin surface begin forming at the deepest layer and work their way up, losing water as they age. By the time the cells reach the surface, they have dried up and their life span is over, a process that takes only about twenty-eight days. These cells are so minute and so numerous that newer cells pushing their way up will slough off old ones at a rate of several million a day.

We help the skin throughout the body by keeping it scrupulously clean so that it can do its job unhampered. For the face, the part of the skin most important to us where beauty is concerned, regular facial treatments are the best way to work with the skin. Facials help to clear away the top layer of dead cell tissue that hides the newer cells lying just underneath, keeping the skin healthy and glowing. Facials also stimulate blood flow to the face and improve the tone of the skin.

Having seen that skin in good condition responds better and heals faster after facial surgery, skin care has become an important adjunct to my medical practice. Facials have been added as a regular part of presurgical and postsurgical procedures. In addition, I have added the remarkable benefits of collagen and other newly developed skin treatments as new weapons in the battle against unwanted signs of age.

Battle is an accurate word, for every day we are all fighting against environmental factors that injure the skin. Extreme cold and biting winds can destroy the skin's small blood vessels as well as bring dryness that accelerates wrinkles. Dry air from indoor heating also robs the skin of moisture. Pollutants in the air—the chemical wastes of industrial plants, exhaust fumes from motor vehicles, and all the other by-products of our technological age—deposit a film of destructive grime on the skin surface and begin to erode its delicate tissues.

While we can combat these irritants by keeping the skin scrupulously clean and generously moisturized, these are enemies to skin beauty that we cannot avoid. Some of the damage that shows up on the skin, however, is self-inflicted. Not taking care of yourself—improper diet, too much alcohol or too many cigarettes, too little sleep, and lack of exercise all leave their mark on the skin, for the general state of the body's health is directly reflected in its outer layer.

By far the most damaging thing we can do to our skin is to overexpose it to the sun. Many of the skin problems I see are a direct result of this overindulgence.

Ninety-nine percent of wrinkling of the skin is a direct result of sun exposure. Sun worship has been going on since prehistoric times. In many cultures, the sun was considered a god, sometimes a malevolent god who was placated only with human sacrifice. In a sense, that is what we are doing today when we bake in the sun, indifferent to the warnings of the irreversible damage that the cumulative effects of the sun can cause in later life. There are many people who draw the blinds to protect their rugs and carpets from sun damage, yet willingly expose their own delicate and irreplaceable skin. Even more distressing are those who pay money to wither their skin in a tanning parlor, or use reflectors to intensify the sun's rays and their damaging effects.

While the glow of a suntan seems to present an image of health, it is actually a reaction by the skin, trying to protect itself from the rays of the sun. Continued exposure to the sun's rays can result in the breakdown of tissue, cellular damage, irregular pigmentation, and degenerative changes in the skin that lead to precancerous and cancerous skin conditions. The need for surgery to remove cancers of the skin is growing at an alarming rate. It is currently the most common of all cancers and has reached epidemic proportions in the United States. From 1930 to 1980 the lifetime incidence of skin cancer has gone from one in every 1,500 people to one in every 150—a tenfold increase.

Protecting your skin against overexposure does not mean that you can never go out in the sun, but it does mean avoiding the most intense hours of sunlight between 10:00 A.M. and 2:00 P.M. and always wearing a protective sunscreen cream or lotion.

Today's sunscreens are rated according to a sun protection factor (SPF) on a scale ranging from two to twenty-three. A preparation with an SPF of two, for example, allows users to stay in the sun twice as long as they could without any protection. The Skin Cancer Foundation and many dermatologists, however, recommend nothing less than an SPF of fifteen, especially on the face.

The ideal sunscreen would screen out both types of the sun's rays, ultraviolet A (UVA) and ultraviolet B (UVB). The

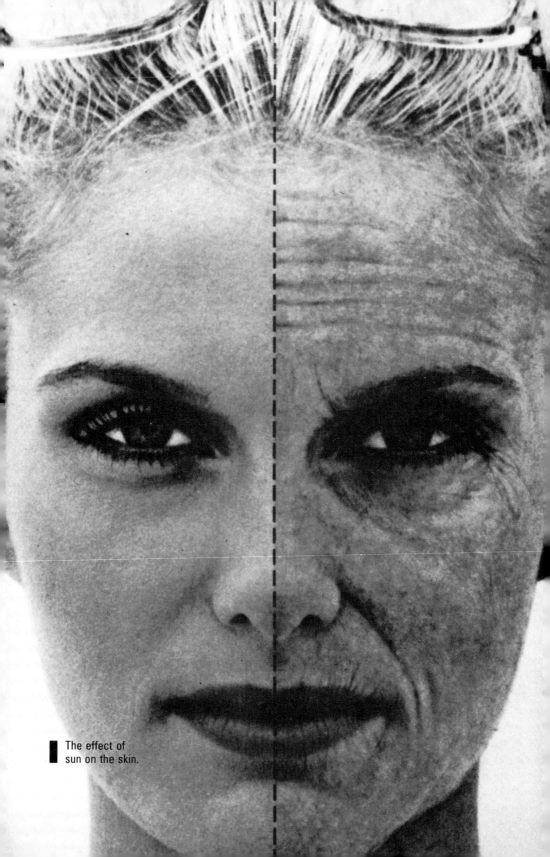

The effect of
sun on the skin.

difference in these rays is in their length. UVA rays are longer and more penetrating. They were formerly thought to be less harmful because they emit less energy, but current consensus is that they can be just as damaging as the UVB rays, which are responsible for sunburn. These not only contribute to skin cancers, but also to the unattractive aging of the skin known as photoaging. Besides harming the body's outer layer, research has shown that high UVB doses can also weaken the immune system, one reason why skin tumors can so easily start on sun-damaged skin and grow into larger tumors. There is some evidence that overexposure to the sun degrades the function of the heart, lungs, and other organs, as well. People who overexpose themselves to the sun look older and are older throughout their bodies.

A protective sunscreen works to protect the skin through a photochemical reaction. The molecules in the substance absorb light and convert it into heat energy. This heat simply dissipates on the skin, but the process is so imperceptible that the dissipation is not felt by the sunscreen wearer. The most effective chemical commonly used is para-aminobenzoic acid (PABA). Remember that sunscreens are not 100 percent effective and that they must be reapplied every few hours, after each swim, and whenever the protective film may have rubbed off or washed away. Makeup preparations containing sunscreens offer more limited protection unless they are opaque or contain 5 percent PABA. Even a minimal sunscreen is better than no protection at all. It is a simple and essential step in maintaining your good looks and your good health.

I should mention briefly here three other skin maladies, common complaints that I often see in consultations about the skin. *Chloasma*, a discoloration of the skin or hyperpigmentation, is often known as "the mask of pregnancy." Its appearance is associated both with pregnancy and with the use of birth control pills. There is no treatment for this condition. While there is no way presently to stop it as a reaction to pregnancy, there is every good reason to be cautious with the use of birth control pills.

Vitiligo, a patchy loss of melanin pigment from the skin is of unknown origin. It usually appears as oval or irregular patches of white skin. This may not be noticeable in winter, but with summer tanning a strong contrast develops, since the area of vitiligo does not tan. This may be helped by judicious exposure to sunlight and by oral medication.

Tinea versicolor is actually a noncontagious disease that causes cosmetic changes in the skin. The typical signs are blotchy patches of varying size and shape ranging in color from whitish to tan to brown. The most striking change caused by this disease is the inability of the affected areas to tan when exposed to sunlight, causing noticeable patches on the skin. Shampooing with a medicated substance is usually effective in treating this malady, though recurrence is common.

It is important to see a doctor when mysterious skin conditions appear since those that are treatable respond to proper treatment most easily when detected early.

ANTIAGING TREATMENTS

Proper skin care will delay the aging process, but even when the skin has been faithfully protected, cleansed, and moisturized, the time inevitably comes when wrinkles and other unwelcome aging signs make their appearance. These are the natural developments that we call *intrinsic aging.* Many of these, such as wrinkling and mottling, are greatly intensified by photoaging, the damage done by exposure to the sun.

The rate of the cell renewal that keeps the skin fresh falls off by 50 percent between the ages of thirty-five and eighty, and the oil glands also slow down their production of sebum over time. Where your skin once glistened from an excess of oil, it may turn dry and dull. This process speeds up with the approach of menopause. Sometimes the surface of the skin becomes rough and leathery.

Since skin layers shed more slowly, they have more time to absorb melanin (pigment) from surrounding tissues, leading to mottling, otherwise known as freckles or liver spots. The formation of growths, both benign and malignant, also increases with age.

The collagen and elastin fibers which give the skin its elasticity and tone begin to degenerate as well, and the skin loses some of its elasticity, the ability to bounce back to its original shape when stretched. This leads to the appearance of fine lines as well as deep furrows in the skin, and the sagging skin and wrinkled neck that make many begin to consider a face-lift.

Problems that were minimal in youth also become more noticeable. Blackheads and broken capillaries may increase in size and number and pores become enlarged.

The aging process begins to be noticeable as early as age thirty. This is when the sagging of the skin commences and the upper eyelids begin to droop slightly. At forty, wrinkles begin to appear on the forehead. Furrows between the eyebrows, excess skin in the lids, and wrinkles at the corner of the eye become more noticeable.

By age fifty, the forehead wrinkles tend to unite to form a continuous line and the furrows are permanent. In the upper eyelid, the skin sags to the proximity of the eye lashes. The corner of the eye develops a downward slope, the nasal tip descends and wrinkles begin in the vicinity of the mouth and the neck.

Age sixty sees a deepening and lengthening of all these changes. The external size of the eye visibly decreases because of the encroachment of the surrounding skin and the wrinkles at the corner of the eye join the line of the bags underneath. By now, a decrease in skin thickness is noticeable and there is marked absence of fatty tissue at the temple and cheek, causing a more sunken look. At seventy, the absence of fatty tissues is even more conspicuous and the descent of the nasal tip more obvious.

Cosmetic surgery can do away with sagging skin, but it cannot erase all of these changes brought on by aging. In fact, by stretching the skin, it may make them more obvious.

But today's cosmetic surgeon has at his or her disposal many new techniques offering a wonderful array of treatments to improve the appearance of aging skin. Some of these, by warding off the effects of aging, may postpone the need for face-lift surgery. Let's look together at the possibilities.

COLLAGEN

The development of expression lines such as deep vertical furrows or frown marks between the brows, and of smile lines, deep lines from the angle of the nose to the mouth or from the mouth to the jawline, are familiar aspects of the aging process for almost everyone. As noted, the first signs are visible on some people even at age thirty.

Injectable collagen is a new substance developed in the last decade that can fill these depressions, taking years off the appearance. It is also an excellent new way to treat acne scars, by filling in the craters.

This collagen should not be confused with cosmetic collagen, an ingredient in many beauty products. Cosmetic collagen is one of nature's most potent moisturizers, but it cannot penetrate the skin to replace tissue.

Natural collagen, a name taken from the Greek word meaning *glue,* is a protein found throughout the body, including skin, bones, tendons, and ligaments. The body's supply is constantly replenished in youth, but as we grow older, the re-

Areas best suited for collagen injections include: wrinkles and deep, vertical furrows between the eyebrows, deep lines between the nose and mouth, wrinkles around the mouth and eyes, as well as furrows in the forehead.

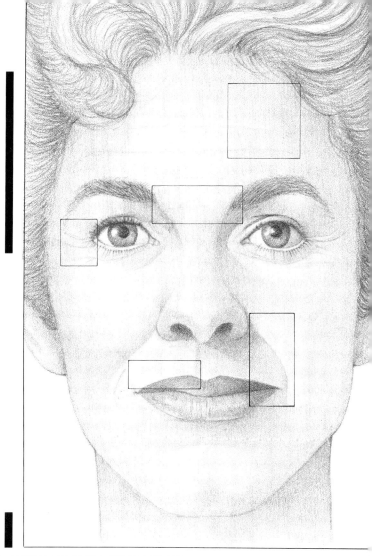

Collagen injection is administered to the postlabial folds.

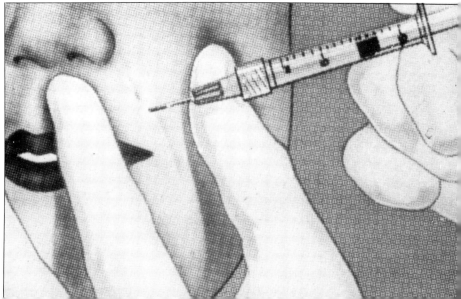

placement process slows down. We lose elasticity and actual tissue.

Since animal and human collagen are very similar, an injectable collagen, a highly purified extract of cowhide, has been formulated that can successfully replace some of the lost tissue in humans. Known as Zyderm or Zyplast collagen, it is so similar to our own collagen that it is readily accepted by the body to replace lost or damaged soft tissue. When injected with a fine needle just below the skin, the collagen quickly meshes with existing tissue, raising indented areas to the level of the surrounding skin. A mild anesthetic is mixed in the collagen solution to ease any discomfort.

For the Zyderm injection to work properly, it is necessary to put in too much collagen, that is to overcorrect the defect because half the substance used is water. This leaves the area looking a little plump for twelve to eighteen hours. In twenty-four hours, the water is absorbed and the area looks normal. No recuperation period is necessary. While the procedure can't be described as fun, in my experience, almost everybody comes back.

Collagen treatments are not for everyone. It is not effective for the deep scars known as "ice pick scars," or for tiny superficial lines such as those often found under the eye.

To be eligible for this treatment, patients must undergo an allergy skin test. Though only 3 to 3.5 percent prove allergic, it is a necessary safeguard. The injections also will not be given to those who are sensitive to lidocaine, the local anesthetic used, or to anyone with a history of extreme allergic response. Other conditions that might prevent the use of collagen are pregnancy, lupus, rheumatoid arthritis, or ulcerative colitis.

Collagen treatments may cost anywhere from three hundred to one thousand dollars, depending on the extensiveness of the area to be treated. Most people require a series of two to three visits, three weeks apart, with touch-ups every six to eighteen months.

When treatments are for acne scars or traumatic defects such as scars caused by an accident, many insurance companies will provide reimbursement.

Collagen treatments are being used today worldwide by cosmetic surgeons and dermatologists who have been individually trained and approved in collagen injection therapy. Over sixty-five hundred physicians in the United States are using it on a routine basis, both for facial defects and self-improvement. More than two hundred thousand patients have been treated with injectable collagen and have been happy with the results.

DERMABRASION AND CHEMICAL PEEL

Once aging sets in, there is no way to restore an unblemished, unlined complexion, but there are two highly effective ways to improve the surface appearance of facial skin that has been wrinkled, roughened, or discolored by the effects of time. This is done by literally removing the superficial layers of the skin, either by abrasion or by using chemicals. While neither of these processes involve incisions, they are definitely medical procedures and must be done in a professional setting by a doctor. Neither is either quick or painless, and in untrained hands, permanent scarring and skin damage can occur.

Dermabrasion, a mechanical scraping of the skin surface, uses a rapidly rotating wire brush or burr to remove the top surface of the skin. A local anesthetic is generally used unless the patient prefers general anesthesia. The face is treated in small sections. When local anesthesia is used, each section of the face being worked on is anesthetized by injecting a medication such as lidocaine that provides a temporary freezing effect lasting for a few hours, long enough for the machine to do its job and the patient to begin her postoperative recovery comfortably. The entire procedure takes from twenty to forty minutes.

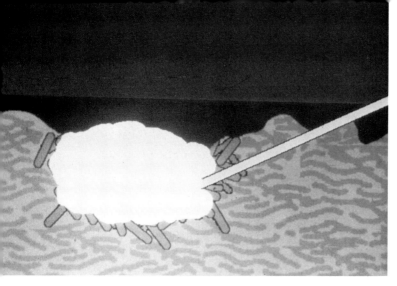

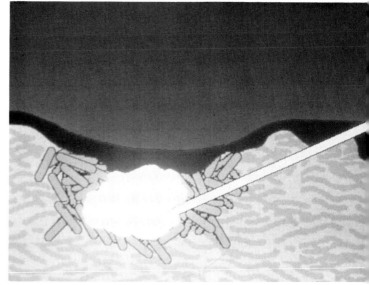

Injectable collagen supplements the body's own collagen, raising depressions to the level of surrounding skin.

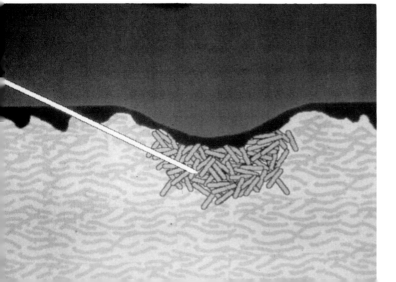

The technique evolved as a means to improve skin scarred and pitted by acne but is also effective for eliminating fine lines and shallow wrinkles and for removing freckles and other surface pigmentations, including premalignant lesions from overexposure to the sun. Deep scars may require more than one treatment. The skin soon regenerates almost entirely, and the procedure can be repeated after a rest period of three to six months.

Chemical peel, also known as *chemabrasion,* is literally the use of chemicals to remove the superficial skin layers. The formula used is phenol in solution with distilled water, croton oil, and liquid soap (Septisol). The solution is applied to the face and an adhesive tape frequently is applied over it. What happens is, in effect, a second-degree burn. After the application, the cauterized tissue remains in place while a new skin is formed beneath it, as opposed to dermabrasion, where the top layers are actually removed. A full facial chemical peel is problematical because even under supposedly controlled circumstances it is difficult to know how deeply the chemical agents are penetrating and the complications can be numerous and serious. Even when used as an adjunct to the face-lift to remove small wrinkles around the eyes and mouth, it can result in depigmentation, with the skin in those areas left lighter than the rest of the face. Because of the high incidence of loss of pigmentation, many women feel they need makeup twenty-four hours a day following the chemical peel in order to conceal the effects of the treatment. While the chemical peel is quite effective, the associated problems should be thoroughly discussed with your doctor before you decide to proceed.

RETIN-A The newest and most exciting development in treatments to reverse signs of skin aging is *retinoic acid* or Retin-A. When Retin-A was first approved by the Federal Drug Administration in the 1970s, it was used as a treatment for acne and it remains the country's leading prescription for acne.

Later, extensive work by Dr. Albert M. Kligman at the Aging Skin Clinic at the University of Pennsylvania School of Medicine showed striking additional benefits for this synthetic derivative of vitamin A. It was found to increase the turnover of the skin cells that normally slows down with aging. As a result of this cell renewal, the outer layer of the skin, the epidermis, becomes thicker and fuller in appearance once again.

Retinoic acid also stimulates collagen synthesis, so that skin furrows even out and fine lines disappear. Applications also increase blood flow and stimulate the formation of new blood vessels. As a result, blood flow improves and the skin takes on a healthier, rosier look.

Further, it was found that topical retinoic acid has significant effects on the texture and characteristics of photoaged skin, skin that has been damaged by exposure to the sun. Retin-A partially reversed or prevented many changes that usually occur in photoaged skin.

Treatment varies according to individual skin types. Normally, Retin-A is applied at night, and a moisturizer is used in the morning. Those with extrasensitive skin might use retinoic acid every other night. The use of moisturizer is essential, since the retinoic acid has a drying effect on the skin. It can also produce some uncomfortable redness and scaling. However, these side effects are temporary, and usually disappear after a month or so. The one caution with the use of Retin-A is that it thins the horny layer of the epidermis, increasing the skin's susceptibility to sunburn. A strong sunscreen must be used whenever the skin is exposed to sunlight.

Research continues on the effects of Retin-A. However, it

has been shown to be safe and effective when properly applied and it is available right now by prescription. For the first time, it gives us the capacity to retard and even reverse some of the changes brought by aging in a simple and safe way. There is every reason to encourage this therapeutic regime as young as age thirty, particularly in young sun worshippers.

No one can stop the hands of time, but with proper care and the aid of some of these new techniques, today it is possible to slow them down considerably.

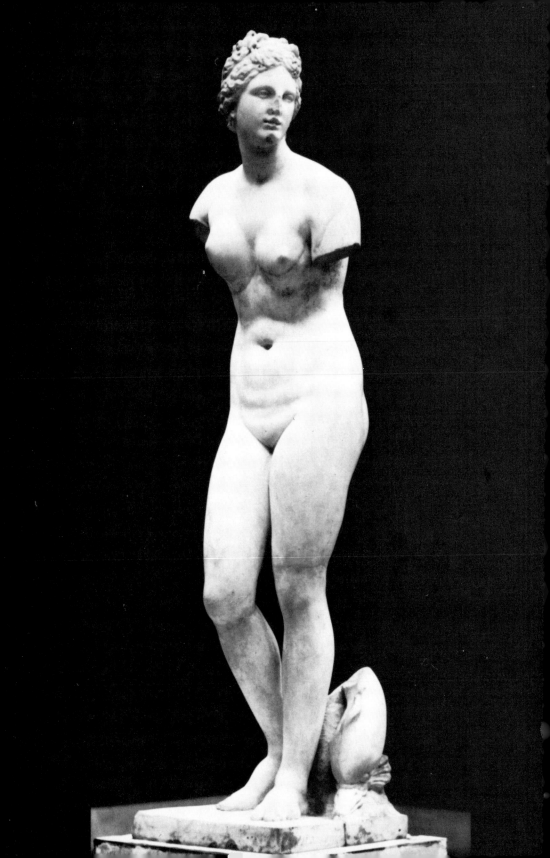

BODY
CONTOURING

PART TWO

INTRODUCTION TO BODY CONTOURING 8

I am convinced that nothing has so marked an influence on the direction of a man's mind as his appearance, and not his appearance itself so much as his conviction that it is attractive or unattractive.

LEO TOLSTOY, *Childhood*

No matter how pleased you may be with your face, the image that looks back at you from the mirror does not stop there.

Many women are self-conscious about certain parts of their bodies, areas so out of proportion that neither diet nor exercise can really change them.

Today, however, it is possible to make changes that will make you happier with your shape. In recent years, the same modern miracles that have transformed cosmetic facial surgery have produced revolutionary new techniques to resculpt many parts of the body.

This is important progress because Americans are becoming increasingly body conscious. Once that meant trying to live up to a movie idol or emulating a perfect 35–25–35 Miss America. Now, as we have become more youth conscious, more active, and more involved in sports and exercise as a nation, many women are less concerned with exact measurements than with having a body that appears trim and in proportion.

This is a healthy trend, because measurements alone have never been an accurate measure of an attractive body. German artist Albrecht Durer expressed well the lack of definitive body measurements when he said, " 'Good' and 'Better' in respect of beauty are not easy to discern, for it would be quite possible to make two different figures, neither conforming with the other, one stouter, the other thinner, and yet we might scarce be able to judge which of the two excelled in beauty."

Few of those who consider the *Venus de Milo* as representative of ideal beauty have actually studied the body contour she represents: slightly over 5 feet tall, 37–27–38 with a 22½-inch thigh, and nearly a 13-inch upper arm. Many a modern woman with such measurements would be seeking help from the nearest spa or fitness center.

The bewildering range of ideals presented through the eyes of predominantly male artists and writers throughout the centuries presents the modern woman with no clear picture of what she ought to look like beyond the current fashion image. This is hardly a reliable gauge. In 1836 Alexander Walker, a London writer, wrote that "excessive leanness is repulsive— nothing can compensate, in women, for the absolute want of plumpness." In the 1960s we had come full circle to Twiggy and a starved unisex shape that led many to extremes of dieting.

Finally, we have recognized that the important thing is not to try to assume someone else's shape but to make the most of the one you have. Body contouring through surgery is one way of achieving this goal. Body contouring is not for everyone. And it definitely is not a substitute for weight control through nutrition and exercise.

But it does offer safe and effective surgical procedures for making positive changes. In the chapters that follow, we will consider the major forms of body contouring; breast reduction and augmentation *(mammaplasty)*, breast reconstruction, stomach surgery *(abdominoplasty)*, surgery of the upper arm, buttocks, and thighs, and the newest highly effective technique for body contouring, *lipolysis*.

Let's look at what is involved in each to see whether they may be right for you.

THE BREASTS 9

*The day is gone, and all its sweets
are gone! Sweet voice, sweet lips, soft hand,
and softer breasts.*

JOHN KEATS, *The Day Is Gone*

The human breast is the only organ of the body to merit two words to describe it—*breast* and *bosom*—each with its own complicated set of connotations and imagery. Such is the importance of the breast to both sexes.

Breast is used most frequently referring to the actual female mammary gland, while bosom is often used to designate the home of nobler human emotions, such as a mother's comforting love and even the final resting place of souls as "in the bosom of Abraham."

The concept of the bosom as the seat of humankind's more noble sentiments was described also by Alexander Pope in his eighteenth-century tribute to the great Roman statesman, Cato:

> *A brave man struggling in the storms of fate,*
> *And greatly falling, with a falling State*
> *While Cato gives his little senate laws,*
> *What bosom beats not in his country's cause?*

Yet despite this romantic imagery, modern women do not often think about their breasts as noble bosoms. Instead, for many women the breasts assume a different but no less important significance. Breasts represent the major physical component of their concept of themselves as women.

One observer of primitive customs and tribal rituals, Desmond Morris, notes that since earliest times, perhaps because the human is the only species of primate having a female with rounded breasts and buttocks, these smooth hemispheres of flesh are the "basic sexual signal of the human female body."

A noted breast surgeon, Dr. John Bostwick III, agrees in his 1983 publication, *Aesthetic and Reconstructive Breast Surgery:* "The breast is a symbol of femininity in our society. It is a source of maternal and sexual feelings and is often the initiating focus of sexual intimacy. Its 'feel,' sensation and appearance nurture the development of a warm, interpersonal relationship."

As a woman and a physician, I know that this emphasis makes the breast an integral part of a woman's sexuality. When a woman perceives something wrong with her breasts, it is not a trivial complaint, but one that should be heard with understanding and compassion.

In an anatomical sense, the breasts are the mammary glands, remarkably designed by nature to fulfill their function of supplying milk for a newborn infant. Beneath the skin of the breast are fatty tissue and lymph vessels, nerves, milk ducts, and glands. The milk ducts open to the nipple, which contains from fifteen to twenty tiny holes that allow a mother to feed her child.

The breast changes through the stages of a woman's life. At birth it is about equal in size for both sexes. During puberty a girl's breast increases to its mature state, mostly through an accumulation of fat and the effect of various hormones in the female body. You need only look around you to see that the breasts develop differently in different women. The size and

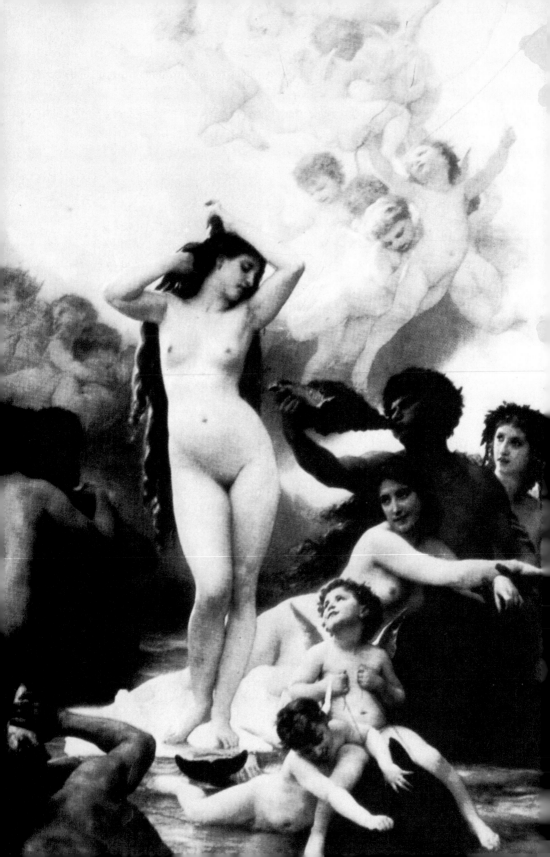

shape are affected by heredity, menstruation, weight gain or loss, pregnancy, hormones, and also by the relentless pull of gravity over time. And women are not always happy with their own lot.

The breasts may not develop sufficiently to make a woman feel physically attractive. Conversely, they may overdevelop to the point where they not only cause embarrassment but actual physical discomfort. While no two breasts are exactly alike, some women have a disturbingly marked disparity in size between their two breasts. And sometimes the breasts lack firmness. They sag in an unattractive way, a condition known as *ptotic* (drooping) breasts. All of these defects can be corrected by today's plastic surgery.

THE DEVELOPMENT OF BREAST SURGERY

The history of breast surgery is an interesting one. In ancient civilizations, external means such as brassieres and corsets, nipple rouge, and nipple rings were used to focus attention to the breasts, and oils and asses' milk were applied to soften and smooth them, but there are no records of surgical procedures to alter the breasts. The ancient Greek healer Hippocrates advised women to sing as loudly as they could to improve the bust line.

It was in 1669 that Will Durston, a layman, wrote for the first time about surgery performed on a big-breasted woman. The first procedure to elevate the ptotic or sagging breast also is believed to have been attempted that same year. The modern procedure known today as *mastopexy* and the first nipple transposition were both recorded in 1911.

Augmentation of the breast by implantation was first attempted by Pierre Fauchard in the mid-sixteenth century. He used as replacement for lost bodily parts such materials as ivory, glass, and paraffin. Credit for the first attempt at modern plastic surgery to deal with defects of the breast goes to Vincenz Czerny, who in 1935 removed a fibroid tumor (a hard benign growth) from the breast of a female patient, filling the void with a lipoma (another type of benign tumor composed of soft fatty tissue) from the same patient.

Silicone was a late nineteenth-century invention, curiously named by a professor at Nottingham University with a word that means uninviting glues. The Dow-Corning Company developed silicone to be used for medical purposes and in 1962 established a Medical Products Division to manufacture and distribute medical quality silicone. During the 1960s many other synthetic materials were tried in augmentation mammaplasty, including acrylic resins, polyethylene foam, polyurethane, and Teflon.

Current breast surgery takes three approaches based on the three major problems encountered in women patients: breasts that are too large, too small, or droopy. Women with marked overdevelopment or underdevelopment of only one breast can be aided either by reduction of one breast or augmentation of the other.

Let's take each problem separately and talk about the corrective procedures for each.

REDUCTION MAMMAPLASTY

Large breasts are problematic for several reasons. From a psychological point of view, they can produce mental anguish in the girl or woman who finds herself constantly regarded as a sex object and subjected to snide comments about her figure.

Buying clothing, a pleasure for many women, is only a dilemma for the large-breasted girl or woman. Blouses and dresses become a means of concealment rather than adornment. Sweaters or abbreviated bathing suits that accentuate the female figure cannot be worn at all.

Younger women are especially vulnerable, sometimes becoming shy and retiring as a result of self-consciousness about their breasts. They may deprive themselves of normal social and athletic activities such as swimming or dancing, which can seem unpleasant, embarrassing, or impossible because of the ungainly appearance and weight of enlarged breasts.

Two research scientists, Goin and Gianini, performed psychological studies on a group of breast reduction patients and concluded that some adolescent patients with large breasts actually viewed their breasts as external handicaps, handicaps that could not be successfully integrated into a positive self-image. I have seen patients who actually block out any idea of the real appearance of their breasts from their consciousness. They are disassociating themselves from a bodily characteristic that feels alien to them.

There are potential physical problems, as well. Poor posture can result from the excessive weight on the chest wall. Pressure from brassiere straps can mean permanent ridging and skin discoloration on the shoulders. If the skin of the breast rubs against the skin of the anterior abdominal wall or chest wall, excessive perspiration may result, causing infection and chronic skin disease known as *intertrigo*. Chronic *mastitis* (painful breasts) can also result from too much breast tissue. And premenstrual symptoms such as shoulder, neck, and upper back pain may be exacerbated by overly large breasts.

Curvature of the spine *(kyphosis)* is another condition that can result when posture shifts to compensate for the weight of enlarged breasts. Abnormal development of the abdomen follows and the belly becomes prominent as well.

If arthritis is a problem, as may be the case with older women, the weight of the breasts on the spine aggravates the condition. Many of my older patients have been referred by orthopedic surgeons, who suggest reduction mammaplasty as a means of alleviating symptoms produced by cervical osteo-arthritis. Plastic surgery does not cure this condition, but removing strain from the spine helps to relieve pain.

BEST CANDIDATES FOR REDUCTION MAMMAPLASTY

There are many sound reasons for considering surgery if the breasts are unusually large. However, as with any surgery, women should be aware of all possible complications before they decide on mammaplasty. Breast surgery inevitably leaves scarring. In some cases, it may also reduce the sensitivity of the breast. And it can make it impossible to breast feed. While the advantages of surgery often far outweigh these factors, a decision should not be reached without learning all the facts in advance.

The ideal patient for reduction mammaplasty is someone otherwise normal in height, weight, and stature. Often women considering breast reduction are overweight. I always advise trying to lose weight before surgery. It makes little sense to restore breasts to a more normal size if the rest of the body is obese and out of proportion. The motivation for further weight loss after surgery is always tremendous. Once the appearance is enhanced, excessive body weight seems even less attractive than before.

Teenage girls are often most eager to do something about the embarrassment of oversized breasts. While youth is no barrier to surgery, it should not be performed until the bra size has stabilized for six months to a year. There is little point in having an operation while the breasts are still growing.

Where breast surgery is concerned, I often find it as important to deal with the attitudes of the patient's family as those of the patient herself. Sometimes young girls who might benefit tremendously from breast reduction meet resistance from their parents. Many teens and young adults tell me that their parents do not know they have come to see me. One recent patient explained that she had discussed her problem with her mother only to be told, "You are being silly and ridiculous. You should thank God that you're healthy and God decided to give you large breasts." She was too ashamed to go to her father with her problem.

I've also seen instances where the mother was understanding but the father balked, saying in effect, "There is absolutely nothing wrong with my daughter. Tell her not to be silly." When parents can be persuaded to talk with the surgeon about their daughter's condition and its possible psychological and physical damage, they often change their minds. I have often had to point out to parents that their daughter's breasts are not normal, something they have a hard time accepting on their own.

In some cases, it is a husband rather than a parent who poses a problem. A husband may not really understand his wife's unhappiness. He states his opposition to surgery by telling her, "I love you just the way you are." Husbands, too, need to understand that while their wives are not freaks, they do have a physical problem that is not normal. It is not a figment of a woman's imagination or a whim like changing the color of her hair. It is a physical problem, one that may not be fatal, but can still do irreparable harm.

If a woman is contemplating pregnancy in the near future, it is wisest to wait for surgery until after she has her baby. The breasts respond to hormonal changes to enlarge during pregnancy. Afterward, involution (reduction in size) of breast tissue takes place, and sagging results that could alter the benefits of surgery. For this reason, I advise married women to have their children before they have the surgery. If a woman hopes to breast feed, there is further reason for postponement.

Some women are unable to nurse an infant after breast surgery.

However, an eighteen-year-old who does not expect to become pregnant for several years need not postpone surgery. It is not sensible to suffer the pains of excessive breast size for that length of time.

One special consideration for a young unmarried woman is the scarring that is unavoidable in breast surgery. She must choose between corrective surgery that will improve her appearance but will leave scars, or living with overlarge breasts. Recently I interviewed a young woman who decided that she preferred her present problem to the scarring, and she postponed consideration of surgery until after she was married. The majority of those I see, however, elect to have surgery— and are happy about their decision afterward.

TECHNIQUES OF REDUCTION MAMMAPLASTY

The breast reduction operation usually is done in a hospital with the patient under general anesthesia unless the correction needed is minimal. The entire procedure takes from three to four hours. Fees range from thirty-five hundred to seven thousand dollars. Since this operation is sometimes performed to relieve physical discomfort, the surgeon's fees and other costs may be partially or even fully paid by insurance. However, if the surgery is elected solely for the sake of appearance, most insurance plans do not offer coverage. The determination is based on the amount of breast tissue removed relative to your body build.

In addition to the usual prohibition about taking any compounds containing aspirin before surgery, women are advised to stop taking birth control pills or other estrogen-containing hormones prior to breast surgery. The breast is the target organ for estrogen, and taking "the pill" or other hormones increases breast size for many women. The surgeon works most effectively on the unchanged normal breast.

Exact techniques may differ slightly from surgeon to surgeon. The most common technique, called brassiere pattern skin reduction, involves both horizontal and vertical incisions that follow the contour of the breast in an inverted T shape from the nipple area down to and within the crease below the breast. The vertical incision includes a circular shaped pattern above the *areola*, the dark pink skin surrounding the nipple, showing where the nipple will be placed on the newly contoured breast.

The surgeon works through the incisions to excise excess tissue, fat, and skin on both sides of the breast. Exactly how much is removed is carefully determined by the patient height and weight, as well as her age and her own wishes. The size of the breasts before surgery is also considered. Many women say to me, "Make me as small as possible," but to take a DD cup down to a B may horrify the patient when the bandages come off. They go from feeling overly endowed to feeling flat-chested.

The contour of the breasts is also important. Enough tissue should remain to maintain the rounded normal form of the breast. I don't find a pancake-shaped breast beautiful, even though some patients do request it.

When the breast is reduced to the proper size and excessive skin removed, the nipple and areola are moved to a new higher location without separating them from their blood supply.

If the breasts are tremendously enlarged, a different technique is used that completely detaches the nipple from the breast before relocating it. This is done only when the surgeon feels it is absolutely necessary since a transplanted nipple loses all sensitivity.

After the nipple is repositioned, skin on both sides of the breast is moved to the midline of the breast and then brought

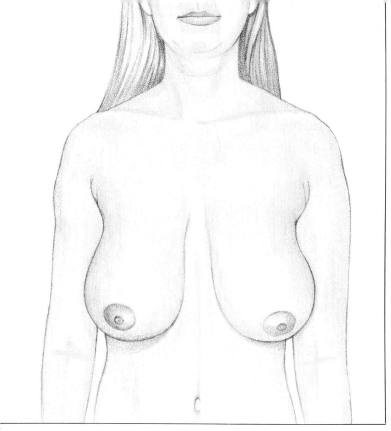

Reduction-
mammaplasty patient,
with oversized, heavy
breasts, before
surgery.

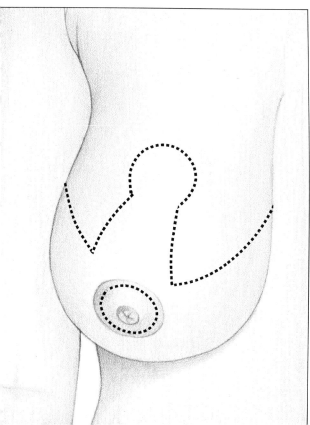

Incisions are made in
the breast to define
the area of excision
and the new
location of the nipple.

Skin located above the
nipple is brought down
and together to reshape
the breast.

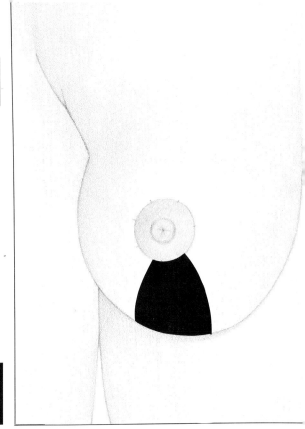

Sutures close the
incision, leaving
permanent scars that are
easily concealed by a
brassiere or bathing suit.

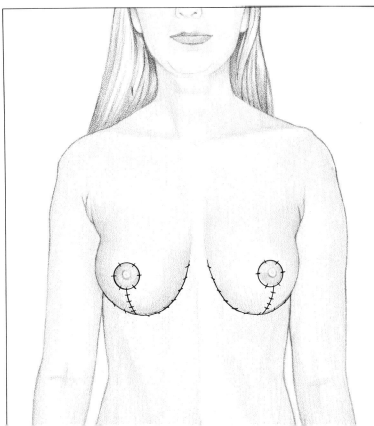

together to recontour the breast. Sutures close the wounds under the breast and around the nipple area. A gauze dressing is then applied to the breasts. I use a "grenadier" dressing, so called because it goes over the shoulders and around the torso, much like the uniform *bandeau* of soldiers in the old grenade regiments.

POSTOPERATIVE CARE

Following surgery, the patient is removed to the recovery room until the effects of the anesthesia have worn off, then returned to her room or, in the case of ambulatory surgery, sent home. Pain is controlled by medication for a day or two and normally then subsides. Hospital patients usually are sent home in two to three days. At this time, or within the first week, any dressing will be replaced by a soft brassiere, which is worn day and night for three to six weeks, except when showering.

Swelling and skin discoloration around the incisions generally will subside in a few days. After surgery, there may be a temporary loss of sensation in the nipples and breast skin. This condition usually improves with time. Sutures are removed within two weeks of surgery.

I allow my patients to shampoo as soon as they feel well enough, even a day after surgery, as long as they have help and can sit in a chair at the sink, taking care to keep the dressing dry. Showers are allowed in a week, when the dressing is removed.

Light activity such as making a meal or going out to the movies can be resumed in a matter of days. Most patients feel well enough to return to work in about ten days. However, as with all surgery, strenuous activity should be avoided for three to six weeks to allow healing. Excessive exercise as well as overhead lifting should be avoided.

Postoperative scars will be visible, but they need not be the cause of anxiety as long as patients are aware in advance that there will be scarring. The most visible scar is the vertical scar from the nipple to the breast fold. When the patient is standing, the horizontal scar will be largely hidden by the breast itself. Neither scar can be seen in low-cut clothing. Scars remain highly visible for about a year, then fade to some degree.

POSSIBLE COMPLICATIONS

Hematoma, bleeding into the operation site, is a possible complication for this and all surgery. Other complications such as delayed healing or infection occur, but only rarely. Infections are treated with antibiotics, draining of the site, and sometimes by local *debridement,* careful surgical excision of infected skin.

Occasionally, poor healing of scars may call for revisional surgery later on.

AFTEREFFECTS OF SURGERY

The younger the patient, the greater the concern about the level of sensitivity of the nipple and the general eroticism that will remain in the breast area following surgery. Erotic sensations of the nipple are often diminished or absent in women who have unusually large breasts, even before surgery. There is some further diminution of sensation around the nipple area afterward, and a complete loss when nipple transplants are called for. Some of this loss may be only temporary, with at least part of the sensation returning over time.

In some cases, especially where nipple transplants are done, there is interference with the ductal system that blocks the egress of milk. This may make it impossible to breast feed an infant following surgery. It is impossible to predict with certainty whether this will occur. However, it is also impossible to predict in advance whether any woman will be able to breast feed. It is a little known and somewhat surprising fact that many extremely large-breasted women produce very little milk. One of the theories concerning this phenomenon is that the weight of the breasts has destroyed the *alveoli,* the glandular portion of the breast, thus rendering the breast incapable of producing milk.

Stretch marks are common in young women with over-enlarged breasts, particularly in the upper portion of the breasts. When the breast is reduced and the skin is tightened, these stretch marks usually become less obvious, but they do not disappear entirely. Only stretch marks of the skin overlying the breast tissue to be excised will be removed completely by the procedure.

PTOSIS; MASTOPEXY

Comedienne Joan Rivers gets a laugh when she jokes about her sagging breasts, announcing, "I wear a 36B—long." But the problem of sagging breasts is not a joking matter for women who suffer from this unattractive condition. Mastopexy, or the breast lift, is the surgical technique used to correct it.

Ptosis or sagging can occur naturally or may be the result of lost volume and elasticity after childbearing. It can happen to small as well as large breasts. In 1976 a Canadian woman plastic surgeon, Dr. Paule Regnault, classified ptosis of the breast into three categories which remain the standard ways of describing this condition today. First-degree or minor ptosis occurs when the nipple is at the level of the fold beneath the breast but above the contour of the breast itself. Second-degree or moderate ptosis means the nipple is below the crease but still above the contour of the breast. In third-degree

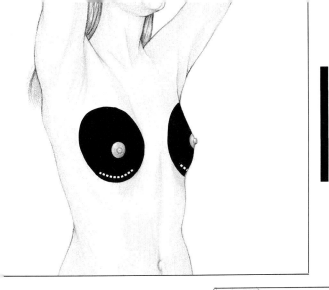

Incisions are made following natural contour lines. Breast tissue or muscle in the shaded area is lifted to form a pocket for the implant.

A cross-section of the breast shows the location of the implant—either in a pocket directly under the breast tissue or underneath the chest muscle.

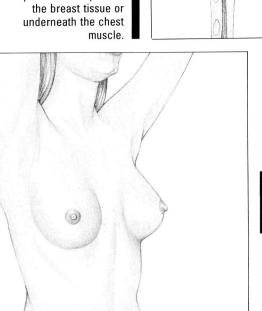

After surgery the breasts are fuller and natural in tone, contour, and appearance.

ptosis, the nipple is below both the fold and the lower contour of the breast.

You can get some idea of your own condition with a simple test. Stand in front of a mirror and find the point of your elbow when your arms are at your sides. Now count up one-third of the way to the shoulder and draw an imaginary line horizontally from that spot across the breast. If the nipple, without a bra, falls below that line, you may have a ptotic breast. A surgeon will use mathematical and geometrical measures both to diagnose and correct the ptosis.

THE TECHNIQUE OF MASTOPEXY

Mastopexy is considered a less major operation than breast reduction, and it may be performed in an ambulatory surgical unit as well as in a hospital. General anesthesia is normally used, though local anesthesia to numb the area around the breasts is an option. The operation normally lasts about two hours. Costs vary from twenty-five hundred to five thousand dollars.

Frequently the breast-lift patient will have a normal-sized breast and require simply a lifting of the drooping breast. This is accomplished by changing the position of the nipple-areola complex (the nipple and the darker circle of skin surrounding it), bringing it up to a more normal position on the chest wall.

The surgeon makes incisions following the natural contour across the breast and around the areola. A keyhole-shaped incision is made above the areola to mark the new location for the nipple. Roughly, the normal position of the nipple is one-third of the way up from the joint of the elbow to the shoulder, when the arms are at rest.

Working through horizontal and vertical incisions, the surgeon removes excess skin from the lower section of the breast. Then the nipple, areola, and underlying breast tissue are moved up. After the nipple is relocated, flaps of skin formerly above and to the sides of it are brought down, around, and together to reshape the breast. Sutures close the wounds under the breast and around the nipple area.

When patients have only minimal sagging, a modified procedure may be used, removing skin only from the areola and the area immediately surrounding it.

Sometimes, when breast augmentation is required, it is performed in conjunction with this kind of lift. When this occurs, the surgeon places a breast implant, or prosthesis, in a pocket created either directly under the breast tissue or underneath the chest wall muscle. Doing both procedures at one time minimizes scarring. Women who are candidates for this double procedure should discuss this option with the surgeon.

POSTOPERATIVE PROCEDURES

At the completion of the surgical procedure, a compressive bulky gauze dressing is placed on the operative site and the patient is placed in the grenadier dressing, as in reduction mammaplasty. The patient is transferred from the operating room to the recovery room, and from there either taken home or back to her hospital room.

This is not a particularly painful operation, but as the patient moves, some discomfort in the area of the excision is normal. Pain-reducing drugs are prescribed for the first twenty-four to forty-eight hours; after that time, they are not usually necessary. If the patient complains of a lot of pain, I suspect a postoperative complication. Many patients go home with only a mild analgesic such as Tylenol or Tylenol with Codeine.

The dressing is changed within the first week after surgery. The wounds are inspected, and nipple-areola complex is checked to be sure that its blood supply is adequate, and the patient is then put into a special brassiere. The bra is worn day and night for three to six weeks following surgery, except in the shower.

The brassiere used in most instances is a sleep bra which is elasticized to give support to the breast. It is a lightweight garment that gives even compression to the breast, not a wired bra nor one that anyone would describe as a harness. It is much like the brassieres that many women choose regularly to wear for sleep.

Some sutures come out within one week. All sutures are removed within two weeks of surgery. Showers may be taken as soon as the dressing is removed. This includes gentle cleansing of the operative site, but care must be taken to pat dry the suture line very gently.

Any stretching, heavy lifting, or athletic activities such as tennis, golf, or swimming must be avoided until six weeks after surgery. Typing and writing usually may be resumed within seven to ten days after surgery. Once again, your doctor will determine the exact time to resume normal activity depending on how quickly the incisions heal.

POSSIBLE COMPLICATIONS

Mastopexy is not a complex operation and there are few complications. As with all surgery, hematoma or bleeding into the operative site is the complication most closely watched for after surgery. If evacuation of excess blood is necessary, it can be done either in the operating room or, if the amount of blood is small, it may simply be drained at the bedside.

If infection occurs, it is treated with drainage and antibiotics.

As in breast reduction, there will be lessened sensitivity in the breast following surgery. A scar around the areola and an inverted T scar will remain after the operation. Sometimes it is necessary to bring these scars away from or toward the midline to conceal them, but this may not be necessary in all cases. The scar will not show when low-cut dresses are worn.

Be aware that scarring, in general, shows lighter than the surrounding skin in Caucasians, darker on black skin. Dark-skinned patients also have the possibility of *keloids,* an over-production of scar tissue. Both whites and blacks may develop thick raised scars known as *hypertrophbic* scarring. Where a hypertrophic scar remains within the confines of the incision, a keloid overgrows the original incision.

Be sure you understand the procedures and the scarring that may follow before you decide on any breast surgery.

AUGMENTATION MAMMAPLASTY

It came as a surprise to me to learn recently about a national survey by a brassiere manufacturer. It showed that by industry standards, 50 percent of American women are flatchested.

Each year, some ninety-five thousand of these women decide to undergo surgery to augment the size of their breasts. Most women who come to me for this elective procedure tell me, "I want this surgery for myself. My husband (or my boyfriend) says I'm crazy, that he loves me the way I am, but I'm not happy with myself." These are the woman I consider good candidates for surgery.

Occasionally, I hear the opposite, however. When a woman tells me that she is not unhappy with her breasts, but her husband or boyfriend is pushing her to have her breasts enlarged, I will not agree to operate. The support of a loved one is important, but it is not a substitute for your own motivation. It is your own desire for change that will make this operation a positive experience.

Medically, small breasts are described as *hypomastia*, a condition in which there is an inadequate volume of breast tissue. This may be genetic or may happen after pregnancy, when involution or shrinking of the breast tissue leaves the breasts smaller than their original size. The same kind of involution may happen in the postmenopausal period.

Size, of course, is relative and what seems adequate to one woman may not seem so to another.

Most of my breast augmentation patients are in their early thirties, but they range anywhere from twenty to fifty. I recently operated on an attractive woman in her midfifties. For the most part, they are not women who are experiencing marital or other difficulties, and are not looking to surgery to solve their problems with the opposite sex. They are women who enjoy an active, competitive "on the go" life-style. They are attractive, have nice figures, are often sports-minded and want to look exceptionally good in a bikini or sports outfit. Many are people in the public eye.

THE TECHNIQUES OF BREAST AUGMENTATION

Breast augmentation is accomplished with implants. It is a procedure that lends itself easily to ambulatory surgery, with the patient going home the same day. The operation takes from one to two hours. Fees are from three to five thousand dollars. A local anesthetic may be used if the implant is placed above the chest muscle; general anesthesia is necessary when the implant is placed below the muscle. However, many patients prefer general anesthesia for this operation regardless of the procedure.

This surgery does not use silicone injections or any type of liquid silicone that may diffuse into the tissues to cause problems. Instead, the silicone prosthesis used today is a removable implant that has proven its safety in use for more than thirty years. Silicone is *nonreactive*, meaning the body is incapable of

130

being allergic to it or rejecting it. Nor is there any instance of it ever causing breast cancer or any breast disease.

The actual implants most frequently used may be any of four types. Three are silicone: a flexible silicone bag containing a silicone gel, a bag of silicone filled with a saline solution, or a combination of the two. A fourth type in current use is made of polyurethane.

Most commonly, the implant is inserted through an incision beneath the breast, but the incision may also be placed in the region of the nipple. After the incision is made, the breast tissue may be lifted up off the muscle or the muscle itself may be lifted. The implant then is placed either beneath the breast tissue or beneath the muscle. The scar is placed in the fold beneath the contour of the breast.

In most cases, I like to insert the implant beneath the muscle. This serves two functions. First, the implant beneath the muscle is harder to detect. The muscle provides more bulk over the implant, producing a softer feeling and more normal looking breast. Second, it is believed that the massaging action of the muscle over the implant may help to produce a softer breast.

Another technique in use is to insert the implant beneath the breast or muscle through an incision in the armpit (*axillae*). I prefer the first approach, which I believe is also the safest, and which results in most instances in a negligible scar, but each surgeon may have his or her own preference.

Some doctors use inflatable silicone bags that expand in place. I do not find these give as good a result as the silicone prosthesis. Also there is a relatively high incidence of deflation of the inflatable bags.

It is possible to combine augmentation mammaplasty with mastopexy when sagging occurs in a very small breast. This dual procedure eliminates the necessity for a T-shaped scar. The incision can be made in the crease below the breast; the breast implant fills out the skin and plumps up the breast.

POSTOPERATIVE CARE

Sterile dressings are placed on the operative site and the patient is placed in the grenadier dressing as in reduction mammaplasty. Normally discomfort is not severe following the operation.

The dressing comes off within one week. The patient is instructed to examine herself beneath the dressing to be sure that the breasts remain soft and that there are no serious problems during the immediate postoperative period. After the dressing and sutures are removed, the wound edges are held together with special sterile adhesive strips and a sleep bra is applied. The bra is worn day and night except for showering for three to six weeks after surgery.

Hair can be washed almost immediately using a chair at the sink, and showers are permitted as soon as the dressing is removed. Normal activity such as typing, light housework, or cooking can be resumed within seven to ten days, but strenuous activity such as swimming, tennis, or golf is to be avoided for three to six weeks after surgery. Intercourse is included among strenuous activities.

POSSIBLE COMPLICATIONS

Once again, while hematoma is not usual, this bleeding into the operative site is the most common of all potential complications.

The wound also could become infected, a particularly troublesome complication with implants because frequently a wound will not heal in the presence of a foreign body. If this occurs, it may be necessary to remove the implant in order to treat the infection. The implant is replaced several weeks later.

Another hazard is the possibility that the patient may stretch or strain, rupturing the incision line. This could result in *dehiscence*, in which the incision separates and the implant actually comes out of the wound. For this reason, special care must be taken to avoid strenuous activity following breast implant surgery.

As in other breast procedures, there may be diminished sensation in the nipple area after surgery.

A final complication is *encapsulation,* which occurs when fibrous or scar tissue forms, completely encircling the breast implant. This is a normal reaction that always occurs, to some degree, but in some people it may cause the breast to become too firm. This can happen on one side or both. There is no agreement as to the cause, but we do know that it is detectable much less frequently when the implant is inserted beneath the muscle. Encapsulation may be helped simply by manual manipulation of the breast to release tension. In severe cases, surgery may be necessary to excise the scar tissue to soften the breast.

OTHER TYPES OF BREAST SURGERY

There are other types of breast abnormalities that can be corrected by plastic surgery. One of these is *amastia,* a very rare total absence of the breast. *Supernumerary* or extra nipples and areolas are common in both men and women. An enlarged nipple may occur on a small breast, as may a small nipple on a very large breast. These may call for simple reduction of the nipple and areola or reduction of the breast, depending on the abnormality.

For every woman over thirty-five, I advise mammograms before any type of breast surgery. Breast cancer is a real and significant threat to the American woman, one that has reached epidemic proportions. Breast reconstruction is an art that is bringing new peace of mind to women who have been deprived of their breasts by cancer surgery, a topic we will discuss more fully in the next chapter.

BREAST RECONSTRUCTION 10

We have a little sister, and she hath no breasts.

"Song of Solomon"

The emotional and physical shock that many women feel when deprived by surgery of their breasts, and the dismay their friends and loved ones often feel at their disfigurement, is hinted at in the poetry of the Bible quoted above. The pitied "little sister" who has no breasts has no womanhood.

Until very recently, the importance to a woman of having two healthy breasts has been misunderstood and even ridiculed in many male attitudes and in the very literature of breast surgery. "You don't really need it" or "It's not necessary for life" are comments I have heard from some insensitive physicians and surgeons, some of whom still regard the breast as just another body gland.

When I was a resident, I found myself being ridiculed by another surgeon because I expressed sympathy for the young patient before us on the operating table, a woman about to undergo a *mastectomy,* surgery to amputate her breast. "I respected you and thought you had more sense than that," he said. "Here you are, chief resident, and what are you so worried about? What's the breast? She's going to live, isn't she?"

Yet a woman's fear and sense of loss at the removal of her breasts is little different from the fear of castration in a male. There are women who, years after surgery, still refuse to look at their chests in the mirror and will not let their husbands touch their flat, scarred chests. They feel mutilated and incomplete. I recommend Betty Rollin's book *First, You Cry* to both men and women who find it hard to comprehend these feelings in women who have undergone mastectomies.

An authority on breast surgery, John Bostwick III, summed up the need for special understanding on the part of all who must help a woman face the ordeal of mastectomy when he wrote, "The woman who develops a cancer of the breast must face simultaneously the significant threat of death and the psychic devastation accompanying complete loss of the breast."

The need for understanding becomes even more urgent when we look at the statistics. Cancer of the breast is the most common malignancy in women (26 percent). Well over one hundred thousand invasive breast cancers are diagnosed every year. The probability that a newborn girl today will develop breast cancer in her lifetime is 9.4 percent, meaning that one in every eleven little girls on average will develop invasive breast cancer. The odds go up if there is a high incidence of the disease within the family. The numbers are a powerful argument to all women for regular self-examination and medical checkups. The sooner the cancer is detected, the less radical the surgery required, and the better the prospect for a successful reconstruction of the breast.

The improvements in recent years in reconstructive surgery have meant new hope for breast cancer victims, many of whom tell me they never feel quite comfortable with an external *prosthesis*, or false breast, that is subject to slipping when a woman is active in sports or dancing. While it can never exactly reproduce the lost breasts, surgery to reconstruct the breast helps restore mastectomy victims' confidence and good feeling about themselves as women.

Plastic surgery for breast reconstruction after mastectomy has been attempted for the past fifty years, but with today's improved breast implants and finer techniques, the chances are significantly improved for a better aesthetic result. Even so, some surgeons remain reluctant to give their patients information about breast reconstruction. Sometimes, perhaps, this is caused by fear of raising false hopes, but other times, as we have noted, it is because of conservatism and lack of understanding of the psychic trauma many woman go through at the loss of their breasts. Every mastectomy patient has a right to full information about the possibility of reconstructive surgery, and her physician has a duty to see that she receives it.

The surgeon who performs a mastectomy has only one goal. It is to save the patient's life by removing the malignant growth in the breast and all the tissue directly or indirectly affected by it. The type of surgery called for determines to a great extent whether reconstructive procedures can be successfully used.

Whenever possible, the treatment of choice today for invasive breast cancer in younger patients is the modified radical mastectomy (also called the Patey procedure, after a British surgeon general). This procedure involves removing the skin and the nipple areolar complex, the underlying gland, and the *pectoralis minor* muscle of the chest. The *pectoralis major* chest muscle is left intact. The lymph nodes (the contents of armpit or axilla) are removed also. This is the technique that leaves the best groundwork for successful reconstruction.

The more radical procedure, called the Halsted mastectomy, sacrifices the pectoralis major muscle and uses an oblique incision excising an area of skin so great that the wound cannot be closed by sutures, but requires skin grafting from another part of the body. It presents special problems to the reconstructive surgeon.

TECHNIQUES OF RECONSTRUCTIVE BREAST SURGERY

Reconstructive surgery aims to restore the normal breast contour as much as is possible, using breast implants. The breasts cannot be restored to a completely normal appearance. The size of the reconstructed breast must often be reduced in order not to overstretch the remaining skin on the chest. The most striking improvement is the psychological one. The natural cleavage between the breasts is restored, which cannot be accomplished with a padded bra. The patient can once again wear low-cut clothes and move actively with confidence. She feels womanly once again.

Many surgeons will perform immediate reconstructive surgery following mastectomy, but this treatment is associated with a higher rate of complications such as bleeding, infection, and even extrusion of the implant. Six months to two years is a recommended waiting period following removal of the breast before reconstruction is begun.

There need be no concern about reconstruction hiding a recurring cancer. There is consensus that if this occurs, it usually does so within the skin, which is not hidden by an implant. If the cancer is in the skin, it can be seen and felt.

Reconstructive surgery can take from two to five hours, depending on the condition of the breast and the type of surgery required. Fees vary similarly, from two to seven thousand dollars.

If there is sufficient skin and underlying chest muscle tissue present to work with, the reconstruction is relatively simple, and may be done on an ambulatory basis. The operation is done by opening the existing scar (or, in some instances, making an incision farther down on the chest wall) and inserting a mammary implant underneath the muscle. The technique and implant are similar to those used in augmentation mammaplasty.

If there is insufficient tissue remaining, more complex procedures are necessary. In this case, the operation is done as an inpatient procedure under general anesthesia in a hospital. This type of reconstruction involves using blocks of tissue from the back consisting of skin and its underlying attached musculature, with the neurovascular supply of blood vessels and nerves kept carefully intact. The technical name for this procedure is the *latissimus dorsi (back) myocutaneous flap*.

In moving the flap, special care is taken not to sever the flap's internal connection to the body's blood supply. This connection or *pedicle* is preserved by carefully moving the flap to its new site through a tunnel created beneath the skin along the side chest wall to the mastectomy site on the front wall. The flap is transferred to its new position without breaking the pedicle connection. The implant is inserted beneath this flap, which is then sutured into place.

Sometimes a flap consisting of skin as well as underlying fatty tissue can be moved up from an obese abdomen and used to fill in the defect, with a breast implant simply placed underneath. A composite flap of skin and underlying muscle tissue from the abdominal area, the *rectus abdomenis flap*, may also be able to be transferred upward, with its blood supply intact, to fill in the defect.

When it is not possible to move a flap with its pedicle intact, free tissue transfer must be done. This requires microvascular surgery to make new connections for the transplanted tissue.

Skin expansion is another approach that may be taken in breast reconstruction. A temporary expander, an empty silicone bag, is placed beneath the tight skin of the front chest wall and is gradually filled with saline solution (salt water) over the course of several weeks. When adequate stretching of the skin has been achieved, the expander is replaced by a permanent breast implant as in augmentation mammaplasty.

There are limits as to how large a breast can be reconstructed. If a very large-breasted woman loses a single breast, reconstruction frequently involves doing a reduction mammaplasty on the remaining breast so that the two will match. The two procedures can be done separately or at the same time.

Similarly, surgery may be indicated if a remaining breast is droopy (ptotic). Since a reconstructed breast is often at a higher position on the chest wall than was originally the case, the drooping breast can be brought up to match it more closely for a symmetrical result. If the ptosis is minimal, it is possible to place the reconstructed breast slightly lower, rather than operate on the second breast.

It should be noted that some surgeons continue to perform the *subcutaneous* mastectomy, a procedure that was in vogue a few years ago. Using this method, the surgeon makes an incision and removes most of the breast but does not remove the overlying skin or nipple-areola complex. An implant is placed beneath the skin or the chest wall muscle. In most instances I do not recommend this procedure. It frequently results in the remaining loose skin wrinkling, puffing, and contracting around the implant, giving the reconstructed breast an unnatural spherical look. An even more important argument against this type of mastectomy is the high risk that cancer will develop in the breast tissue beneath the nipple area and in other breast tissue that may be left behind.

Reconstruction of the nipple

The nipple-areola complex can be reconstructed at the same time as the breast reconstruction or as a delayed procedure. There is an advantage to doing these operations separately. If the two are done in one operation, it is sometimes difficult to get one nipple positioned to exactly match the other. It is easier to match and make the two nipples symmetrical after the wound has healed and the breast has settled down into its permanent position on the chest wall. When the operation is done in two stages, the nipple-areola complex is created six to twelve weeks after the initial reconstruction to allow for this healing to occur.

The areola, the rosy area around the nipple, can be reconstructed in a variety of ways. The surgeon attempts to match the natural skin whenever possible. For patients whose areola is pink, a skin graft is usually taken from behind the ear. If the color is a deep pink or brown, the inner thigh may be used. When the area is very dark, a graft may even be taken from the *labia minora*, the tissue near the vaginal opening.

The surgeon has a number of options also in rebuilding the nipple. A small wedge of skin and fat may be removed from the ear lobule as a graft or the skin and fat from the ball of the fourth toe may be used. The reconstructed nipple projection cannot be the same as a natural nipple, but there is at least an elevation of tissue that simulates a normal nipple-areola complex.

POSTOPERATIVE CARE

When all the incisions have been sutured closed, the patient is removed to the recovery room until effects of anesthesia have worn off, then returned to her room, or, in the case of simpler surgery, allowed to go home. The length of hospitalization varies according to the type of surgery done. In more complicated procedures, the wound must be drained, so the patient might have to remain longer until the drainage decreases significantly enough so that the tubes can be removed. An average total stay for this more complex procedure is five days.

Bulky dressings are placed on the wounds initially. Later, a soft brassiere is worn day and night, except when showering, for three to six weeks.

The amount of pain following surgery also depends on the type of procedure done. The more complicated the surgery, the more discomfort. When necessary, narcotics are prescribed to ease the pain. Simpler procedures typically require less medication. As with most operations on the skin, the discomfort does not persist for a long period of time.

Some sutures come out within one week, all are removed within two weeks. Once the dressings are removed, it is safe to bathe or shower, taking care to be very gentle with the surgical area. Hair can be shampooed as soon as the patient feels well enough, as long as no undue strain is placed on the operative site and the arms are not raised overhead.

There may be a loss of sensation in the breast area following surgery, but this is usually temporary. The nerve endings frequently regenerate and regain their sensitivity.

As in other surgical procedures, the patient is advised to avoid strenuous activity for three to six weeks. Special care must be taken to avoid any strain from stretching. Pulling on the operative area raises the risk of wound dehiscence. When the incision comes apart and the implant is exposed, infection becomes a real danger. Infections do not usually heal around a foreign body, so if infection occurs, it is often necessary to remove the implant to permit the infection to heal and the inflammation to subside. Another operation is then required to replace the implant. It is obvious that this is a situation to be avoided, and that postoperative care on the patient's part is important.

Sexual intercourse also is to be avoided for three to six

weeks, and the newly reconstructed breast should not be manipulated during this time.

POSSIBLE COMPLICATIONS

Besides the above-mentioned risk of infection, there is the usual surgical risk of hematoma, or bleeding into the operative site, requiring the evacuation of blood and control of the bleeding.

A very serious complication may occur if radiation treatments administered after a mastectomy have compromised the blood supply. This can jeopardize the success of the operation, resulting in partial or total loss of the flap. Additional surgery, skin grafting, and the removal of the implant may be required.

Scarring can be extensive from this type of surgery. The woman undergoing breast reconstruction begins her surgery with a significant scar from her mastectomy. If enough tissue remains, it is usually possible simply to open that scar and insert the implant. Depending on the location of the scar, however, sometimes it is preferable to make a new incision lower on the chest wall or near the junction of the chest and the abdominal wall, creating a new scar.

If the flap procedure is used, the scarring on the chest is much more extensive. The donor site or area from which the flap was taken, most often the back, will also bear a scar. It can be either oblique or vertical, according to the doctor and the patient's preference. A back scar can usually be placed in such a way that it is covered by a bathing suit or sundress.

If a composite block of tissue is taken, meaning both skin and underlying muscle, an elliptical scar will result on the area reconstructed.

Some women worry that the presence of scar tissue means they will not have sensation in their breasts. However, areas adjacent to scars do not lose their sensitivity, even though the scar itself lacks nerve supply.

Breast reconstruction cannot restore a premastectomy breast nor can it be done without producing scars, but for many women this is a small sacrifice compared to the mutilation they felt before it was performed.

It is an operation that restores more than a part of the body; it gives back the precious feeling of being a whole woman again.

THE ABDOMEN **11**

By any name—*abdomen, belly,* or *stomach,* or by the less dignified common terms of *pot* or *gut*—the part of the frontal anatomy located between the thorax and pelvis has always come in for more than its share of attention.

The Bible tells us in Psalm 101 that ancient people used to read character not only in facial characteristics, but in stomachs: "Whoso hath also a proud look and high stomach: I will not suffer him."

For many years an ample belly also was considered a sign of prosperity, as noted by Shakespeare in his "Ages of Man" speech:

> *and then the justice;*
> *In fair round belly with good*
> *capon lin'd*

144

In Shakespeare's time as in our own, however, a growing abdomen had another, less welcome meaning. When he wrote,

> *Have you not a moist eye,*
> *a dry hand, a yellow cheek,*
> *a white beard, a decreasing leg,*
> *an increasing belly?*
> *Henry IV, Part II*

Shakespeare was referring to the "increasing belly" that comes to many people with the passing years, an unwelcome sign of age.

There is a difference, however, between those who develop the common malady known as middle age spread, and those who have a real deformity of the stomach area and a weakening of the abdominal wall. An overblown belly (the term comes from the same old English word that gave us *bellows*) can be a particular problem for the female, who has an innate tendency to a rounded stomach. One of the more interesting anatomical differences between the male and female form is that the female belly is naturally convex or round, while the male abdomen is concave. While artists and poets have extolled this difference, celebrating the beauty of the rounded female form, if the belly actually begins to bulge, there are few of either sex who find it attractive.

Losing a large amount of weight may account for sagging skin of the abdomen. Pregnancy also often causes an unflattering change in a woman's body by loosening the muscles of the front of the abdominal wall and destroying the elastic fibers of the skin that keep the belly firm. This produces sagging and a general lack of healthy firmness in the abdominal area.

Many young mothers mistakenly believe that they can remedy this condition by exercise after the baby is born. Muscle tone may be restored, but where the elastic fibers of the skin have been damaged, producing stretch marks, skin tone and resiliency cannot be restored.

Early surgical techniques to correct deformities of the abdominal wall date only from the 1890s, so abdominoplasty, less formally known as the tummy tuck, is a modern phenomenon. At first, surgeons in France and Germany used this procedure to correct functional problems associated with hernias and very large, pendulous bellies. In 1899 an American surgeon named Kelly first used the term *abdominal lipectomy* to describe the technique he later used on eight patients at Johns Hopkins University, a technique recognized as being an important psychological as well as surgical breakthrough for patients with abdominal deformity.

BEST CANDIDATES FOR ABDOMINO-PLASTY

Most of the women I see who are considering a tummy tuck have developed a sagging stomach either as the result of pregnancy or the loss of a large amount of weight. Occasionally, I have also seen girls in their early teens who are not fat, but because of hormones at puberty have grown so rapidly that they developed stretched-out skin making them look as though they had had several children.

It is an operation that I have performed on housewives and executives as well as go-go dancers. It is appropriate for anyone who is concerned with her appearance, especially in abbreviated clothing or bathing suits. In most cases, the woman is not obese, but simply has a lax or mushy abdominal wall.

It should be noted that not every woman who has children needs abdominoplasty. Some women are blessed genetically and may look even better after several children than others who have no children but have not taken care of themselves. Some can go through several childbirths and emerge without even developing stretch marks on the stomach.

Others who are distressed at a new "potbelly" following childbirth are looking at the wrong procedure to correct it. If the abdominal wall itself has not been damaged, diet and exercise may be the best prescription for excess weight, or the new procedure of lipolysis, discussed in chapter 13, may be the best way to get rid of a small amount of excess fat. The surgeon's examination will be able to pinpoint the cause of the sagging and determine whether surgery is in order.

Abdominoplasty also can be a corrective for the rarer condition called an "abdominal apron," which is occasionally seen in very obese persons. This occurs when the skin of the front abdominal wall stretches out and folds down over the thighs, sometimes even to the knees, resembling an apron of skin. The entire apron may be removed by surgery.

However, it should be understood that a tummy tuck is not "a little tuck here and a little tuck there," but a very extensive operation. A candidate must be in good health or the procedure cannot be done.

It must also be understood that this is an operation that results in scarring, even though the surgeon will attempt to camouflage the scarring as artistically as possible and locate the scars where they cannot be seen when a bathing suit is worn.

As a side benefit, the tummy tuck operation can do away with prior scars from a cesarean section or appendectomy and with many stretch marks. During the procedure, the surgeon can also move scars from earlier surgery such as a gallbladder operation to a lower location where they will be less conspicuous.

Abdominoplasty is not advisable for a young woman who has had one child and plans to have more. Subsequent pregnancies will simply repeat the stretching process that destroyed elasticity and resulted in sagging of the abdominal wall. It is wiser to wait until no further children are planned.

Age is not a barrier to surgery. A teenager who has lost a large amount of weight and experienced unattractive stretching of the abdominal wall might want to consider surgery, even knowing it might have to be repeated later on.

There are also many older women who were unaware of their surgical options when sagging occurred after childbirth and who have always been bothered by their excessive "potbelly" and flaccid skin of the abdominal wall. Many of these women elect to have this procedure in their fifties or even later. As long as the general health is good, there is no reason not to consider a procedure that improves the psychological well-being as well as the appearance.

As with other plastic procedures, I always caution any woman considering a tummy tuck not to expect the surgery to solve problems that stem from other sources. Recently, I saw a woman of twenty-three who had quickly had several children and now wanted a tummy tuck. The condition of her abdomen looked fine to me and I told her so. Her answer was, "It's not the body I had before my children, and I'm ashamed to show myself to my husband." I felt in this case I would do her a great disservice if I were to operate without her consulting a psychologist or psychiatrist.

TECHNIQUES OF ABDOMINO-PLASTY

The tummy tuck or abdominoplasty operation always is done in a hospital because of the potential for a large amount of bleeding during surgery and the need for careful postoperative care. Because of the bleeding, it is particularly important for the patient to avoid aspirin or any aspirin-containing products for ten days before the operation. Aspirin interferes with blood clotting and makes it more difficult to stop bleeding.

General anesthesia is required. The procedure usually takes from three to four hours, with fees ranging from thirty-five hundred to seven thousand dollars.

For the most aesthetic result, the scar must easily be concealed under a bathing suit, which means that in most cases vertical scars will be made. To accomplish this, surgeons have developed a fine technique known as the W-plasty, so called because it leaves a scar in a gentle curve resembling the shape of the letter W. The scar is placed running from side to side across the lower portion of the abdomen, the area known as the *suprapubic region.*

Some surgeons ask their patients to shave the hair in the pubic area a few days before entering the hospital, so that the hairline is obvious at the time of the operation. I have not found it necessary to shave patients at all. Many studies actually indicate that the incidence of infection is higher if you do shave. In either case, a bath with disinfectant soap is prescribed the day before surgery.

To obtain the best results markings are made on the patient in the standing position according to very careful measurements determined by the surgeon.

A surgical marking pen is used in order to draw a W whose center is located above the pubic hair. The limbs of the W extend downward and sideways into the area of the inguinal fold, the fold where the leg and torso meet. The line then follows this fold slightly upward to each side. This drawing forms the W shape. Lines are then drawn from the ends of the W up to the navel or belly button to help in centering the incisions and final location of the belly button.

After the patient is placed on the operating table, further markings are made on the stomach, beginning at the ends of the W and extending upward above the navel to the rib area. This outlines for the surgeon the area where a flap of skin and underlying fat will be raised from the underlying musculature, a procedure known as undermining.

The lower incision then is made and the flap of skin and fat is raised. At the belly button, a circular incision is made around the navel so that the flap can be moved up without

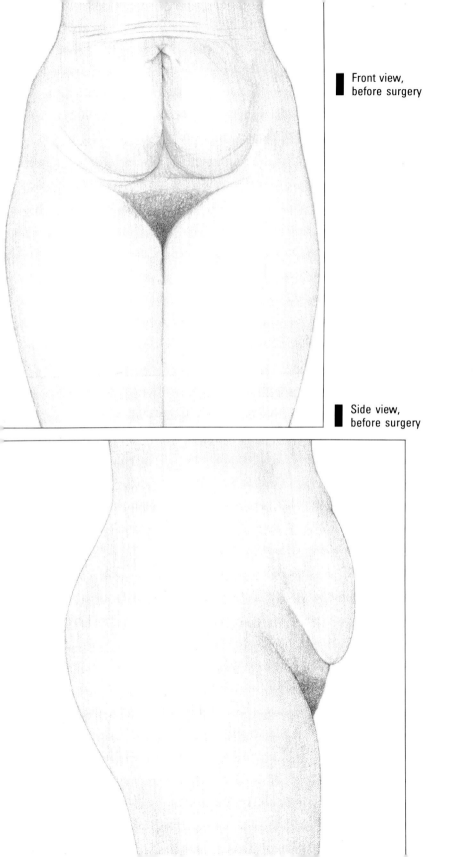

Front view,
before surgery

Side view,
before surgery

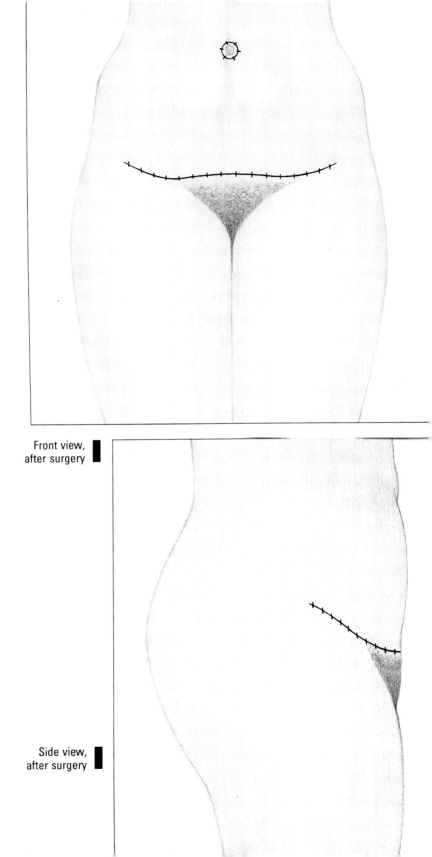

Front view,
after surgery

Side view,
after surgery

detaching the navel from the pedicle or stem of tissue that connects it to its blood supply.

The excess abdominal tissue consisting of skin and fat is then removed. The operating table is gently angled into a position that bends the body, flexing the legs slightly so that the wound can be closed without tension. The proper position for the new umbilical site is carefully determined on the reduced stomach. A small elliptical excision of skin is done at this site on the skin flap so that the navel can be brought through and stitched to the surrounding skin edges. The resulting scar blends with the existing umbilical scar and is not noticeable.

Stretch marks and previous scars from a cesarean section or appendectomy may often be removed with the excised skin and gallbladder or other scars located higher up on the abdomen may be brought down below waist level so that they can be hidden by abbreviated clothing. Midline scars above the belly button seldom can be moved all the way down to the bikini line.

There is a related procedure that may be done at the same time as the tummy tuck. The *rectus abdominus* muscles—the muscles responsible for the tone and strength of a portion of the abdominal wall—are located at the midline, one on the right, the other on the left, and are very close together. They extend downward from the rib cage to the pubic area. When a woman has had children, there is a tendency for these muscles to become separated, producing a clinical condition known as *diastasis recti*. The surgeon can often detect this condition by feeling the area during an examination of the abdomen. While the surgeon is performing a tummy tuck, the covering over the muscles is exposed and may be sewn together to make it stronger, giving added support to the abdominal wall.

Scars from an abdominoplasty are greater if there are conditions that the W-plasty technique cannot correct. If the patient is very obese, with excess skin both horizontally and vertically, a different procedure must be used. A horizontal incision is needed to get rid of the fat roll that lies low down on the belly, while a vertical incision is required to remove the remaining fatty excess in that direction. The final result from that incision is a T-shaped scar from the incision that is known as a fleur-de-lis.

For those who have lost an unusually large amount of weight—sometimes one hundred pounds or more—a belt lipectomy may be necessary to remove the abundance of flaccid skin left hanging on the newly thin frame. This incision goes completely around the body at waist level. Though the scar is extensive, many find it is far preferable to a lifetime of stuffing excess skin into a pair of pants or a girdle, almost like an overblouse.

After the wounds are closed, a dressing is applied over the suture lines. A large amount of gauze and soft padding are placed over the whole undermined area and held in place by surgical tape. Later, the patient will maintain gentle pressure over the operative site by wearing supportive undergarments.

POSTOPERATIVE CARE

The patient is taken to the recovery room following surgery until the effects of anesthesia have worn off, then transferred to her own room. Two drains are placed deeply in the surgical area, brought out through small incisions in the pubic area where the pubic hair will hide the resultant scars. The drains are necessary because of the large area of dead space that remains where undermining has been done. This area produces fluid that takes a long time to get back into the circulatory system. Without drainage, there is the possibility that it might build up causing a condition known as *seroma*, with the danger of infection developing. The drains are removed as healing progresses.

General anesthesia often causes postoperative nausea. As

with all major surgery, the patient is kept on a liquid diet until regular food can be tolerated. If surgery is done at 8:00 A.M., the patient usually is having clear liquids such as ginger ale or tea by 2:00 or 3:00 P.M. Most are back on a near-normal diet by dinnertime, all by the following morning.

The patient cannot straighten up immediately after surgery without danger of pulling the suture line apart or interfering with the flow of blood to the lower portion of the flap, resulting in possible loss of tissue in that area. She remains in bed for up to twenty-four hours following surgery, on her side resting in the fetal position, with feet tucked up, or when on her back using pillows propped under the knees to take the tension off the suture line. For two weeks afterward she is instructed not to straighten fully, but to walk in a bent over position that will not strain the suture line. This is a temporary discomfort that is well worthwhile to ensure a smooth recovery.

A catheter may or may not be needed to draw the urine from the bladder. I usually try to discover whether or not the patient can void on her own. If she cannot, either because of the position in bed or because of the location of the incision, a catheter may be inserted. It is removed once she is out of bed usually within twenty-four to forty-eight hours postoperatively.

Postoperative pain varies in intensity from one patient to another. Oral medication is prescribed for moderate pain, intramuscular for more severe discomfort. I should note for the record that intramuscular injections are not popular. They hurt!

Patients are allowed out of bed on the first day after surgery. On the second or third day the drains come out. The dressing is usually removed within a week after surgery, and showering is then permitted. The patient is discharged on the third or fourth hospital day to continue recovery at home, gradually relaxing the bent over posture as the incision heals.

154

The doctor usually sees the patient to remove sutures and any remaining dressing in one week. All sutures are removed by the fourteenth day after surgery. Then periodic visits are scheduled until the healing is at a stable point, within six months to a year. I usually send patients off to resume their normal lives within six weeks after surgery, with the reassurance the scar will continue to fade as more months pass.

Patients are advised to wear some type of gentle supportive garment such as elasticized panties or panty hose with tummy control for four to six weeks after surgery.

Exposure to the sun should be carefully avoided for several months. A sunburn on an area that has recently been operated on to create a flap can further compromise blood supply to that region and produce serious complications. As long as the scar remains immature and pink, it should also be carefully protected with sun block or sunscreen; otherwise it could become permanently pigmented.

Following abdominoplasty, normal activities should be resumed slowly, varying with each patient's recovery rate. Among my patients, I have met stoics who say to me, after one week, "There is nothing wrong with me. I feel great," and others who are still complaining after six weeks.

Activities such as driving a car or returning to a desk job can be resumed usually within two to three weeks. Strenuous activity such as golf, tennis, or jogging should not be undertaken for at least six weeks after surgery.

The good results of the tummy tuck are permanent, unless a patient has a child or gains a great deal of weight after surgery, stretching the abdominal skin once again. If this occurs, the incision can be reopened and some of the extra skin excised.

POSSIBLE COMPLICATIONS

Severe pain in the immediate postoperative period might indicate the presence of bleeding and hematoma formation at the surgical site. When this occurs, the patient must be returned to surgery and the wound reopened so that the bleeding can be controlled. The wound is then closed again.

Infection is possible with any type of surgery, but I have not found this a common occurrence with the tummy tuck.

If the wounds are closed under too much tension, the blood supply could be compromised, but if the patient is careful not to straighten up too soon, straining the sutures, healing usually will run smoothly.

Scar formation also is normal with surgery. If hypertrophic scars or keloids occur, scars that are typically raised and reddish in color, they may be injected with cortisone that will soften the scars, causing them to flatten and lighten in color.

The operation is *extraperitoneal*, meaning the surgeon does not have to go into the *peritoneum*, the internal cavity that contains such organs as the gallbladder, intestines, and liver, unless there are unusual circumstances such as the discovery of a hernia, a weakness in the peritoneal lining which may allow an organ or a loop of bowel to poke through to the outside. Sometimes the surgeon may also find a loop of bowel caught up in a scar from previous surgery such as an appendectomy. In thin patients, hernias may be detected in presurgical examinations; in more obese women, fat may mask the hernia. Either way, if a hernia is present, it is necessary to open the peritoneum to repair it, introducing the possibility for an *ileus*, a paralysis of the bowel, to develop. Such patients will not be allowed food after surgery but will be placed on intravenous feeding until normal bowel sounds begin. This is a rare occurrence.

A tummy tuck is major surgery and is not to be undertaken on a whim. But for those who have been plagued with an unattractive accumulation of fat in the belly area, recontouring to a smooth firm stomach can make a world of difference in shape as well as in self-confidence.

There are other areas where body contouring may be able to correct troublesome conditions. Let's look at what can be done for unsightly bulges of the thighs, buttocks, and arms.

THE THIGHS, BUTTOCKS, AND ARMS 12

Am I not fallen away vilely since this lact action? do I not bate? do I not dwindle? Why, my skin hangs about me like an old lady's loose gown . . .

SHAKESPEARE, *Henry IV, Part I*

F alstaff's complaint has been echoed by countless women.

Some of these women have abnormal deposits of fat in certain areas—usually the buttocks, thighs, or arms—that cause unaesthetic bulging, spoiling an otherwise good figure and normal appearance.

Others have lost a tremendous amount of weight, and though they are now considered thin, find they have great folds of skin hanging down around certain parts of their bodies.

These unattractive excesses cannot be changed by diet or exercise. Deformities in the proportion of thighs, buttocks, or arms to the rest of the body will yield only to plastic surgery, including the newly developed suction technique called lipolysis, which we will discuss in detail in the next chapter.

Like the breasts, the buttocks and thighs assume special

importance because they are important elements in the erotic life of a woman, a fact evident by their emphasis in the arts.

Traditionally, the thighs have been related to fruitfulness and hence to sexual activity. From 1934 until recent times, the Hays Code, guardian of public morals in motion pictures, forbade the showing on camera of a woman's inner thigh, the last cinematic bastion of feminine modesty.

The emphasis on a woman's buttocks can be seen in ancient statuary which often gave them exaggerated prominence. A woman's buttocks do normally protrude more than a male's, a characteristic that many men find very pleasing, indeed. Anthropologists have noted that where this trait is abnormally pronounced, as among women of certain tribes of southern Africa such as the Hottentots, Bushmen, and Bantu, it is to the delight of their men. Charles Darwin thought this so remarkable that he described the condition (today called *steatopygia*) in some detail. "It is well known that with many Hottentot women, the posterior part of the body projects in a wonderful manner. This peculiarity is greatly admired by the men."

Darwin also quotes his contemporary, Sir Richard Burton, as reporting that the men of Somaliland, a people of mixed Mediterranean and negroid stock, "chose their wives by ranging them in a line and by picking her out who projects farthest *a tergo* (behind)."

The Victorian bustle was an example of a more recent attempt to replicate a look that was considered pleasing to males.

However, times have changed and so has our ideal of the physical form. By any name—"bum," "tush," "derriere," "fanny," or "rump"—today's woman is often embarrassed if her buttocks area is out of proportion. And in the abbreviated sports clothes and slacks of our day, oversize thighs are far more noticeable than when they were hidden by the long full skirts of earlier generations.

The problem of oversize thighs and buttocks was addressed

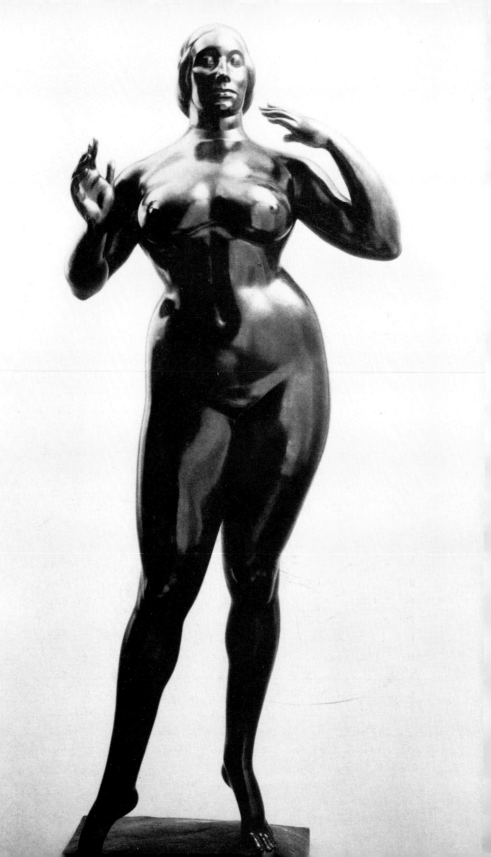

by plastic surgeons for the first time in the 1950s. Surgery for obesity of the thigh area was reported in 1952, and in 1954 the modern procedure for correction of oversize buttocks was developed. Similar techniques may be used when the upper arm is greatly oversized, making it difficult to wear normal clothing. While this type of surgery has been revolutionized and greatly improved through lipolysis, it is still worthwhile for comparison to look at the older standard procedures for each of these areas.

TECHNIQUES FOR BODY CONTOUR SURGERY

Body contour surgery in all areas usually requires the excision of both fat and overlying excess skin. This type of surgery is generally performed in a hospital under general anesthesia because the areas operated on are extensive and a great amount of tissue is removed, and may include significant fluid loss. This does not necessarily mean a blood transfusion will be required, but adequate intravenous fluid replacement is essential during surgery. Only the arm procedure is occasionally done on an ambulatory basis.

Because of the large area to be operated on in thigh and buttock surgery it is especially important that patients avoid aspirin in any form for at least ten days before the operation is scheduled. Prior to surgery, in the privacy of an examining room, surgical markings are made to guide the surgeon in placing the incisions. Since flexing the hip or assuming a normal sitting position should be avoided for two weeks following surgery, the patient is given instruction in getting out of bed using the "log roll" technique, keeping hips and knees straight.

The surgery varies in time from four to five hours, depending on the location of the operation and the amount of tissue to be removed. Fees also vary, anywhere from four to seven thou-

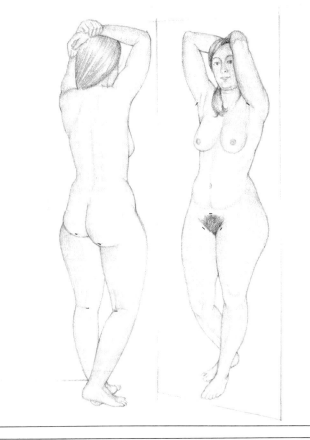

Before surgery
short incisions
are made
through the skin
to introduce the
instrument that
will remove fat
in the shaded
areas.

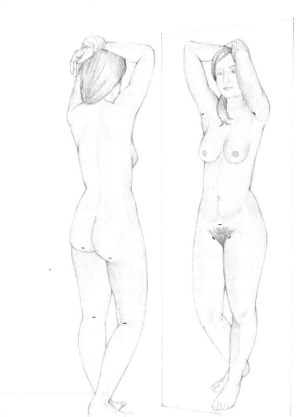

Sutures close
the small
incisions,
leaving no con-
spicuous scars.

sand dollars, according to the complexity of the procedure required.

Thigh surgery

Corrective thigh surgery may be required on the lateral thigh, the inside upper thigh, or the hip area, depending on the type of problem.

When the fat deposit is in the area of the lateral thigh (not quite as high as the hip), the condition is commonly known as the "riding breech" deformity, because the body's contour is similar in shape to jodhpurs or riding breeches that stick out at that portion of the upper thigh. I prefer another term, *violin deformity*, which more clearly pictures the three components of this condition, the hip, an indentation or hollow just below, and then the bulge of fat in the area of the thigh. To remove the excess fat and overlying skin, the incision begins laterally on the thigh, extending into the buttock crease and toward the midline into the vaginal area. The resultant scar is very long and while the surgeon strives for a thin scar, it sometimes stretches out and becomes wider than either doctor or patient like to see.

Another problem with this traditional method is that the force of gravity and the action of the underlying muscle frequently cause a scar that is originally placed inconspicuously in the buttock crease to be pulled down onto the leg, ending on the upper rear thigh. It is then clearly visible with brief clothing such as shorts.

Because the scarring from this procedure is marked and excessive, many plastic surgeons prefer not to perform this operation, fearing they will be creating a deformity as bad as the one they are correcting. As we will see, lipolysis now can correct this problem with only miniscule scarring. Only in rare cases when the fat deposit is so massive that excess folds of skin would remain after lipolysis is this procedure usually considered today.

To correct a bulging inside upper thigh, it is necessary once again to remove both underlying fat and excess overlying skin. Although the operation prevents the chafing that results when bulging thighs rub together, it also leaves a disfiguring scar that runs down the midline of the thigh from the groin area to just above the knee, either in a straight line or a series of gentle curves. The operation is rarely done unless the condition is a true physical problem because the scar from this procedure often is almost as unsightly as the problem that has been corrected.

When hips are the problem area, whether lipolysis or direct excision is indicated depends on the amount of fat present as well as the age of the patient. From the surgical point of view, key considerations are the location of the resultant scar and its final appearance. Surgical procedures need only be considered for the thigh area today in extreme cases, morbid obesity for example, since moderate amounts of fatty deposit can easily be suctioned off through lipolysis.

Arm reduction

Excision of fat or hanging skin in the arm from the axilla, or armpit, to the elbow is usually indicated for a patient who has either a large amount of hanging skin on the upper arm or simply an enormous arm. Either condition makes it difficult to wear normal clothing on the upper body. In some cases the woman cannot fit her arm into the sleeves of blouses or dresses, in others the fleshiness is so prominent that she is embarrassed to wear short-sleeved clothes.

Most typically, deformity in the arm results either from the aging process in a heavy person or in a younger individual who has lost a large amount of weight. In either case, a great fold of hanging skin is the result.

To remove excess skin, the incision is located on the inside upper arm from the axilla (armpit) to above the elbow. The scar could be either a straight line or a gentle series of curves. Because the scar will be large and visible, this procedure also is done only when there is a real and obvious deformity.

Buttock lift

A procedure simply to lift the buttock without excising fat is not feasible. In order to firm the buttocks, fat and skin must be excised, with the suture line placed in the buttock crease to make the scar as inconspicuous as possible.

The buttock lift frequently is combined with the operation for the "riding breech" or "violin" deformity of the upper thigh. The surgery then involves a tightening of the whole backside.

However, a scar in the buttock crease frequently is pulled down on the leg by the force of gravity. When this occurs, it is extremely difficult to retain the firm buttock that is most pleasing to the eye.

This is an appropriate spot to mention that while some women have an overabundance of fat in the buttocks area, others are so flat that they feel their figures are unattractive as a result. In some cases, this is a congenital defect in which the muscles have not developed properly. It is possible to augment the buttock with implants, but it is a problem area because you are introducing a foreign body that is being repeatedly traumatized every time the person sits down. For that reason, this operation is not recommended or performed frequently. It would be called for only in case of a very serious deformity.

POSTOPERATIVE CARE

Following the closing of the incisions with sutures, dressings are applied and the patient is removed to the recovery room until the effects of anesthesia have worn off. If a hospital stay is indicated, the patient will then be returned to her room. The "violin" or "riding breech" surgery requires hospitalization for several days. For other types of body contour surgery, however, while bed rest is prescribed for twenty-four hours following surgery, the patient may go home to rest in her own bed. The plastic surgeon decides on the best course for each patient's condition.

Frequently, when the thighs are operated on, drains are placed in the wounds. These are usually left in place for two or three days after surgery. The reason for this is the considerable dead space left after tissue is removed and while healing takes place. This area contains fluid lost to the circulatory system. Without the drains, excessive fluid accumulation would cause the condition known as seroma, and the danger of an associated infection.

The surgical dressings are left in place for several days following surgery. The wounds are usually inspected within three or four days after surgery. Stitches are removed within one to two weeks, depending on the type of closure used.

Driving or any strenuous activity is not permitted for three to six weeks following thigh or buttock surgery. Arm surgery may be less restrictive, depending on how quickly healing takes place. It is important to avoid any trauma to the operated area, including so-called ordinary household accidents. I still vividly recall a woman I saw during my residency who had gone grocery shopping two weeks after surgery. She had fallen with her bag of groceries and the trauma caused the previously excellent results to be ripped apart. It is only sensible to observe restrictions during this brief postoperative period. The time will go very quickly if you occupy it visiting with friends and planning what you will do when your attractively contoured body has healed.

POSSIBLE COMPLICATIONS

Many of the same complications mentioned in preceding chapters could apply to body contouring as well: excessive bleeding (hematoma), excessive body fluid accumulation (seroma), and wound infection that would require treatment with antibiotics and drainage. Displacement of the buttocks crease scar onto the leg or thickening of the scar (hypertrophy) are also possibilities. Loss of feeling in the skin surrounding the incision may also occur in this type of surgery, as with any procedure in which a large incision produces a significant scar.

But by far what should be considered most here is the scarring itself. Body contour surgery is a trade-off, removing unattractive bulges but leaving a prominent scar. It is major surgery that should not be undertaken lightly, but carefully considered in consultation with a plastic surgeon.

For some, the answer may well be lipolysis, one of the major advances in plastic surgery techniques. Let's look now at how this breakthrough improves prospects for those considering body contour surgery.

LIPOLYSIS 13

He that will not apply new remedies must expect new evils, for time is the greatest innovator.

FRANCIS BACON

Ever since the modern discovery that the lines of the human body could be improved and deformities corrected by the art of the plastic surgeon, everyone has hoped for new techniques to aid the surgeon in his or her role as body sculptor—techniques that would minimize the pain and risk and scarring that are attendant with any surgical procedure.

Within the last five years a remarkable European technique called lipolysis (from *lipectomy* and *hydrolysis*) or suction surgery has produced most welcome results in our own country and around the world. Although research and evaluation of lipolysis are ongoing, and conservative approaches are still advised, many surgeons who have been exposed to the technique believe it represents a significant advance in body contour surgery. Read on to learn why more Americans, male and female, are opting to have this procedure done when they meet the qualifications—and why some cosmetic surgeons, myself included, prefer lipolysis to traditional surgical methods when the patient's condition offers the option to choose this newer method.

In simplest terms, lipolysis uses suction to remove localized deposits of excess fat. It may be used in the thigh and hip areas, for buttocks and arms, for moderate fat deposits in the abdomen, and even for double chins.

The basic procedure involves making a very small incision in the skin, usually camouflaged in a natural body crease, then inserting a slim instrument called a *cannula* (from the Latin word *canna* or reed), a flexible tube attached to a suction unit that is used to draw off fatty cells. One of the major benefits is the tiny incision which reduces scarring to a minimum.

A variety of names have been associated with this technique: fat suction, suction lipectomy, suction curettage, lipolysis aspiration, or the Illouz technique. I use the term *lipolysis* given by Dr. Yves-Gerard Illouz, a pioneer in its development. Dr. Illouz, a Frenchman, has performed this procedure over ten thousand times since he first announced his method in 1976.

Earlier methods required loosening the fatty tissues before suction by scraping with a curette, the same type of instrument used in a uterine dilation and curettage, or D and C, the common operation to scrape clean the lining of the uterus. This method was developed in the mid-1960s by Dr. Josef Shrudde of Cologne, West Germany. By the mid-1970s, Dr. Uerick Kesselring of Lausanne, Switzerland, was using the procedure to help young patients with moderate cases of the "riding breech" or "violin" bulge of the outer thigh.

In 1976 in Paris Dr. Illouz developed an improved instrument, the blunt cannula, and, rather than curettage, used a special solution which was injected to break up the fatty deposits.

Because the announcements and demonstrations of suction methods generated so much interest and controversy among surgeons and the public, in 1982 the American Society of Plastic and Reconstructive Surgeons directed a team of fourteen plastic surgeons to visit the pioneer clinics in Switzerland, Germany, and France and take a closer, critical look at both the Kesselring (sharp undermining) and Illouz (blunt cannulation) techniques. This committee of respected professionals reported back to the larger membership of the society in January 1983. While their report recommends caution, suction lipectomy was found to be a satisfactory method of removing localized fat deposits in certain cases when used by "appropriately trained and experienced surgeons." The report stressed the importance of eye-hand coordination in performing this technique, a judgment once rendered more poetically by a sixteenth-century writer, "In a good surgeon, a hawk's eye, a lion's heart, and a lady's hand" (Display of Dutie).

Here are some of the findings issued by the committee in their January 1983 report:

1. Lipolysis is not a treatment for general obesity, nor is it a substitute for diet and exercise.
2. The suction technique is most satisfactory on persons under forty or those having good skin elasticity.
3. The technique is effective in the hands of trained and experienced surgeons, but in the hands of untrained practitioners could lead to disastrous results.
4. Plastic surgeons experienced in body contouring should have no difficulty in learning the technique by a combination of observation, symposium, and clinical hands-on operative experience.

Since this is a relatively new technique in the United States, the society has been helping to educate the profession by sponsoring seminars in the proper use of lipolysis. It has also issued public warnings against abuse of lipolysis by untrained persons. It cannot be stressed too many times that lipolysis is surgery, not a procedure to be taken casually or to have performed in a beauty salon or spa. The seeming simplicity of this procedure has attracted many who do not understand its serious implications or choose to ignore them for their own gain. Anyone electing this particular type of surgery should be doubly sure that the surgeon is board certified in plastic surgery and professionally trained in this new technique.

CANDIDATES FOR LIPOLYSIS

In the past, when a patient requested surgical body contouring, careful preoperative counseling was required to explain that eliminating one deformity could create another in the extensive scarring left by surgery, particularly in the "riding breech" operation. Often, after detailed explanations, the mutual doctor-patient decision was to live with the deformity rather than the scars.

Today, lipolysis offers the benefits of surgery without the scars, and I readily suggest it for my patients who meet the criteria for suction lipectomy.

Let's take a closer look at who is a good candidate and the reasons for the criteria laid down by the surgeons' committee.

Since the skin is not cut and trimmed in lipolysis as in traditional body contour surgery, skin elasticity is essential in order for the skin to contract and conform to the new form created after fatty deposits are suctioned away. For that reason, most agree that the procedure works best in younger persons—under age forty. Yet, many people over forty whose skin retains good elasticity have had the operation done with good results. It is also possible for skin-tightening procedures to be used effectively with lipolysis. The experienced surgeon is the best final judge of whether the condition of the skin is appropriate and whether follow-up surgery is necessary or desirable.

This is a procedure intended for someone of reasonably normal weight whose localized fat deposits distort an otherwise normal contour. It is not recommended for very obese people because there is a limit to the amount of fat that can be siphoned off safely. Even in cases where the procedure is repeated, it cannot produce an overall reduction of fat, but rather concentrates in small areas. Nor will lipolysis take away the fat condition popularly called *cellulite*, which shows up as dimpling of the skin.

Those who have observed the remarkable results of this newer procedure have noted most of all the psychological exhilaration of patients returning for their checkups two to three weeks after the operation. The response has been positive and encouraging. After lipolysis, women whose abnormal depositions of fat have resisted dieting or exercise have happily reported to me that they are able to fit into jeans and slacks comfortably for the first time in their lives. Others, after a lifetime of buying tops of one size and bottoms a size or two larger report wearing clothing normally for the first time—and even buying clothes a size or two smaller. And, there is no trade-off in unsightly scars.

LIPOLYSIS TECHNIQUES The procedure may last from forty-five minutes to two hours or more, and fees range from three to six thousand dollars, with an additional one thousand to fifteen hundred dollars added if more than one area is treated. A local anesthesia can be used when small areas are involved; when excess fat deposits are extensive general anesthesia is administered. In some cases, a short stay in the hospital may be indi-

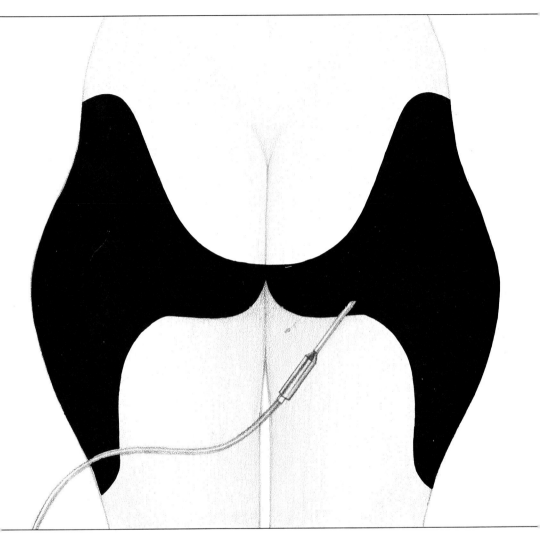

A long hollow tube, open at both ends, is inserted and the fat is suctioned out of the body by using a vacuum.

cated, from one to two days depending on the area operated on and the extent of fat removed.

The tiny incisions required, about one-half inch in length, are just enough to accommodate the hollow tube or cannula, and can be virtually hidden in the buttock crease for many individuals, whether surgery is for thigh, buttock, or hips. Through this one small slit, the inflexible tube used can be long enough to be manipulated carefully from the point of incision to reach the hip or buttocks, and down the leg all the way to the knees for many patients. Others may require separate incisions, depending on the doctor's judgment as to the most beneficial procedure. For the abdomen, the incision can be made in the leg crease near the pubic area, around the belly button, or in the pubic hair. Double chins may also be treated, with an incision made behind the hairline. The armpit area is frequently the choice for an incision to reach fat deposits in the arm.

There are two lipolysis techniques in current use, wet and dry. In the trained hands of an experienced plastic surgeon, they are equally effective. The choice is left to the discretion of the surgeon, and may well rest on his or her expertise with each technique.

The dry technique involves inserting the instrument, then suctioning off, at one atmosphere of pressure, the unwanted fatty cells. (For the nonphysicist, an atmosphere is a unit of pressure equal to the pressure of the air at sea level, or approximately 14.7 pounds to the square inch.)

The wet technique calls for injecting a solution of sterile salt water and an enzyme called *hyaluronidase*. Hyaluronidase splits and lowers the viscosity or thickness of *hyaluronic acid*, a substance that is present in body fluids and that acts as the cement holding internal tissue together. A fifteen-minute period is allowed to pass after the injection before the instrument is inserted. The suction is then turned on and the fatty tissue deposits, now easier to remove, are sucked out through plastic tubing into collection bottles.

Care must be taken not to remove more body fluid than the body can compensate for. As mentioned, if there is too much fat to be withdrawn, the procedure is done in two steps. The patient is sent home to heal from the first lipolysis, and may return later—often within six to eight weeks—to repeat the procedure.

Only a few sutures are needed to close the incisions, leaving inconspicuous and usually well-concealed scars.

POSTOPERATIVE CARE

Immediately after removal of the instrument and termination of the procedure, elastic dressings are applied to compress the area treated. These snug elastic dressings, called "splinting," sweep upward, fighting gravity and helping to prevent sagging. They promote skin shrinkage to conform smoothly to the new shape the surgeon has created. The initial dressings remain in place for about three days. Sometimes a long-length, corsetlike garment may be used to secure firm compression of the area and to reduce swelling and skin discoloration. Some doctors also suggest wearing a long-legged girdle regularly for one to two months after the dressing is removed.

The patient is brought to the recovery room until the effects of anesthesia wear off, then returned to her room or taken home. After surgery, some pain may be present for several days. Medication will be prescribed to keep the patient comfortable.

The patient is up and about in a day but exertion is restricted during the entire first week. The decision on when to return to work depends on the individual degree of swelling and discomfort. Normally, lipolysis patients are back to normal routine within one week. They may resume strenuous activity in three to six weeks.

The hair may be shampooed in a basin any time after the surgery, but the patient is not allowed to shower until the dressings are removed. Driving is permitted whenever it is comfortable for the patient and when restriction of movement has eased.

POSSIBLE COMPLICATIONS

The procedure has minimal complications from bleeding or infection. However, rippling, dimpling, or sagging of the skin over the treated area can occur. Patients who are overweight have a greater possibility of contour irregularity and poor skin redraping. An older individual with loss of skin elasticity may require surgical removal of excess skin as a secondary procedure to achieve maximum results.

The ad hoc committee of fourteen surgeons who evaluated lipolysis in 1983 pointed out that in the five-year period from 1977 to 1982, results from the procedure showed not one report of embolism (blood clot), damage to the veins, or loss of overlying skin. They noted two advantages of this technique, the fact that perforating (deep) vessels were not injured by blunt cannulation, and that there was no damage to the diffuse network of tissue connecting the overlying skin to the tissue beneath the skin. The evaluating team concluded, "The committee unanimously agrees that suction lipectomy by the Illouz blunt cannula method is a surgical procedure that is effective and safe in trained and experienced hands and offers benefits which heretofore have not been available."

As lipolyis is studied more widely and used by more Americans, it is only natural that the questions raised about traditional methods of body contouring by plastic surgery should be raised in this newer context. Why would a woman (or man) want to undergo lipolysis treatment for localized fat deposits if the rest of the body is normal, even beautiful? Why risk any surgical treatment at all, when the rest of your body is "as perfect as God could give anyone"? These are questions that my patients, too, have often heard from concerned family members and friends. They are questions I would like to discuss with you before our consultation ends.

But first I would like to take time out for a chapter on the men in your life and what cosmetic surgery may do for them.

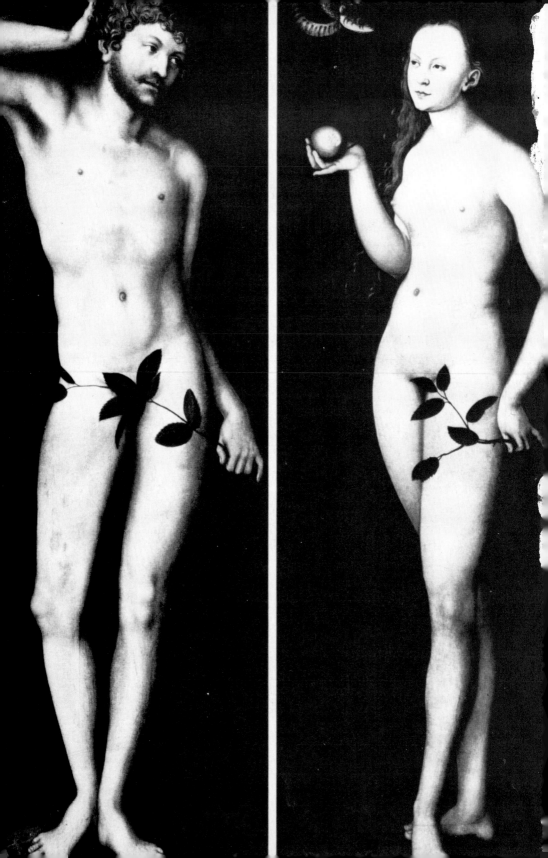

SOME ADDITIONAL CONSIDERATIONS

PART THREE

COSMETIC SURGERY FOR THE MAN IN YOUR LIFE 14

Whenever two people meet, there are really six people present. There is each man as he sees himself, each man as the other person sees him, and each man as he really is.

WILLIAM JAMES

A s a woman I feel empathy for the special concerns of women, but as a plastic surgeon I am well aware that a man's self-image and peace of mind are equally important. Men are no less worried about appearance or about signs of aging than women are—they simply tend to talk about it less.

Women have had the advantage of an early start and good press in making cosmetic surgery more acceptable and accessible. They have also been more willing to take action to make changes in themselves.

Logically, however, in a society that puts a high premium on youth and fitness for both sexes, it was only a matter of time until men would catch on and begin to seek the same benefits that women have been enjoying from cosmetic surgery. As Spanish playwright Lope de Vega put it so aptly, "Man is the powder, woman the spark." In a recent survey on men over age thirty-five, two-thirds of those polled approved of a man having a medical procedure to combat the signs of aging for reasons of either career advancement or simply for self-esteem.

So, like most surgeons today, I am seeing a dramatic increase in male consultations. A third of my patients today are men. Male doctors and lawyers, public figures, and private citizens alike are feeling more comfortable about seeking to make themselves look better, often with the encouragement of a supportive wife or woman friend. In fact, it is no longer unusual for husband and wife to come in together for consultations. One couple I saw recently came initially to talk about a face-lift for the wife and eyelid surgery for the husband. When he saw the good results of his wife's operation, the husband returned to schedule a face-lift of his own.

You, too, can lend information and moral support to your own male candidate for cosmetic surgery. Basic techniques for male procedures are similar to those outlined in the earlier chapters of this book. In this chapter, we will look briefly at some of the differences for the male patient, and discuss fully a problem that disturbs many men, male pattern baldness.

It is worth noting that there is nothing new about men seeking to improve their looks. They are following a precedent that dates back to ancient times. The plumage of the male bird and the body coloration of many male animals have always been more showy than the female, a fact that ancient peoples often mirrored in their cultures. Body paint was used liberally by many tribesmen to show rank and status. Egyptian kings and princes took their cosmetic paint pots and pencils with them to the grave. And cultures not so ancient also exhibit colorful plumage of the male in elegant costumes and powdered wigs.

Some male adornments came about by accident. For example, when Louis XIII lost his hair and beard because of the sudden onset of disease, all the socially acceptable males immediately began to wear perukes (small wigs) like the king's. The fashion spread throughout the Western world.

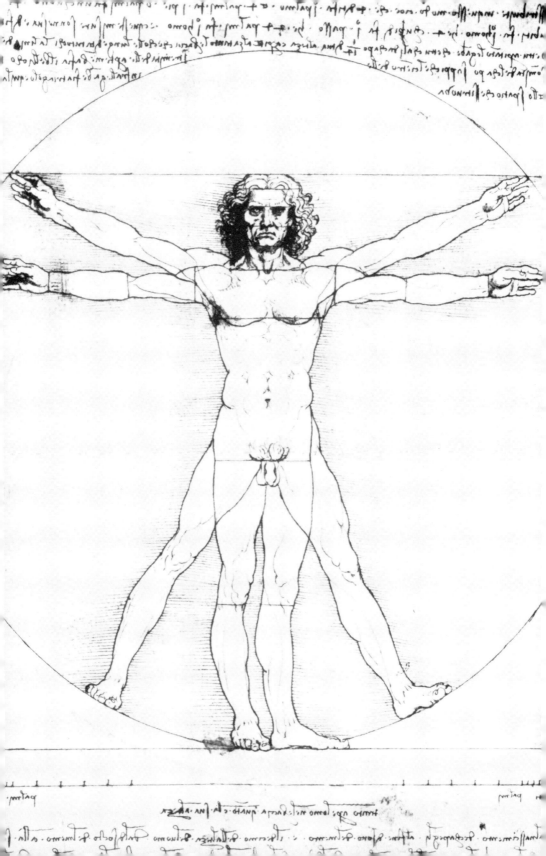

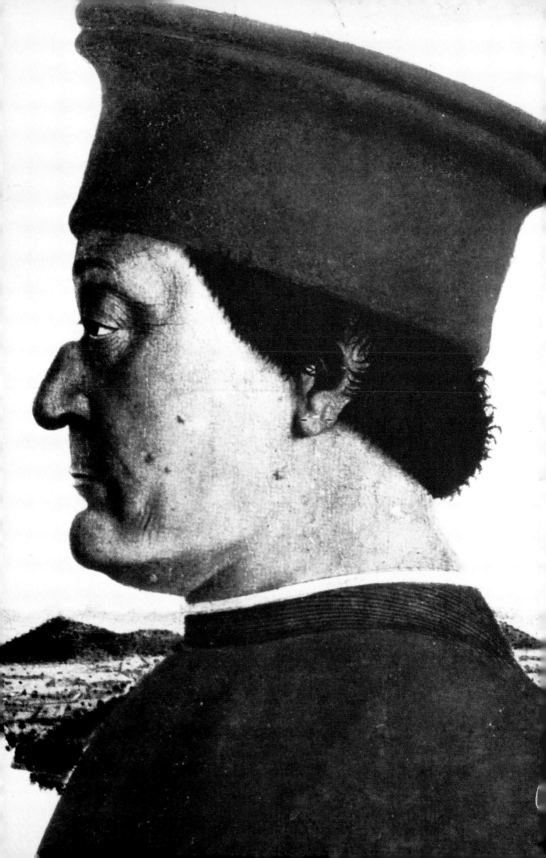

In the early 1800s men like the dandy Beau Brummell were the very picture of male sartorial splendor, but Brummell's death in 1840 did not end male interest in finery. During the long reign of Queen Victoria, it was the male of the species, not the female, who was entitled to maintain a beauty kit consisting of a rouge of perfumed chalk for the face, castor oil and beeswax for the hair and beard, and tweezer for the eyebrows. At the same time a well-bred woman's skin remained pallid. The only "painted women" of this period were prostitutes.

Just as has been true for women, the ideal of male beauty or handsomeness is often in the eye of the beholder, and it has changed markedly with the times. The well-dressed man of the eighteenth century, with his corseted figure, padded chest, powdered wig, and enameled face, would be very much out of place in the 1980s.

Today's American male ideal is firm of jaw and wide of chin with clear eyes, a strong mouth, Roman or large nose, and stylishly groomed hair. Above all, he projects a picture of vigor, fitness, and youth. Never has it seemed more important for middle-aged executives to take five or ten years off a face that still has years of leadership capacity ahead. Baggy eyelids and sagging skin may be perceived as signs of dissipation, not a desirable image in an age when many executives have switched from martinis to Perrier and spend hours jogging or working out on Nautilus machines.

It is not surprising that blepharoplasty (eyelid surgery) is the most requested procedure by men. The face-lift, too, is growing in popularity. Those who elect surgery often are reacting to Bennett Cerf's observation, "Middle age is when your old classmates are so gray and wrinkled and bald they don't recognize you." The men who seek cosmetic changes want to feel better about themselves in the presence of peers, male or female, and more confident when they spy their own reflection in passing a shop window. I have seen car salesmen and truck drivers as well as company presidents take on the self-confidence of much younger men after facial surgery.

The way was paved for some men by seeing the good results of reconstructive facial surgery that prominent public figures like Jason Robards, Mark Hamill, and Van Johnson displayed following automobile accidents. In the film *Raintree County*, fans of Montgomery Clift may still observe the famous Clift face before and after plastic surgery for a severe wound that cut from his nose through his upper lip. Stars like Henry Fonda, Jean-Pierre Aumont, and Dean Martin also show facial scars, and they have been vocal in their gratitude for correction of defects that could have damaged their careers.

Many other prominent men in the public eye, including politicians, have benefited from visiting image consultants, who help them change their dress, hairstyles, and speaking manner to make a more pleasing public appearance. A visit to a cosmetic surgeon is a logical next step in image enhancement.

I find that many men need even more careful psychological screening than my women patients. Some are subject to a macho image that makes them embarrassed and reluctant to admit they want help. It is also important to be sure they have a realistic idea of the scarring they can expect from surgery. Even more vital is insuring that male patients understand what surgery can and cannot do for them. It is unlikely that a facelift, a changed nose, or even a restored head of hair will bring back a lost love or win a promotion that is not deserved. As with women, the best male candidate for surgery is someone who is not looking for the fountain of youth or a magic formula for success, but who simply wants to look his very best for as long as he can. The best result from plastic surgery is not a transformation into a new person, but enhancement of your own looks in order to feel better about yourself.

The majority of male cosmetic surgery candidates present one of the following complaints:

- nose too prominent
- aging face
- baggy eyelids
- baldness
- head and jaw out of proportion
- breasts enlarged
- Adam's apple too prominent

The surgical techniques to correct most of these defects are basically the same as have been described earlier. Let's take a brief look at some of the special considerations each procedure may entail from the male point of view:

Facial surgery

Face-lift and eyelid surgery techniques on the male face are very similar to those for women. Male patients require careful monitoring during the procedure as well as in the immediate postoperative procedure. The difference in male and female hormones makes for a difference in skin quality. Where estrogens cause thinning in a woman's skin, male androgens produce thicker and oilier skin. Because of their facial hair, males also have increased *facial vascularity,* meaning more blood vessels in the face to support the hair's growth. This gives them a greater tendency to bleed during facial surgery.

An important consideration to many men is that the lifting and stretching of the facial skin in a face-lift affects the appearance of sideburns. Usually, there is a space between the ear and the hair. This space may be decreased or even eliminated completely in an extensive face-lift that pulls the hairy portion closer to the ear.

The beard will be affected also. In the face-lift procedure, some of the bearded area of the face is pulled back behind the

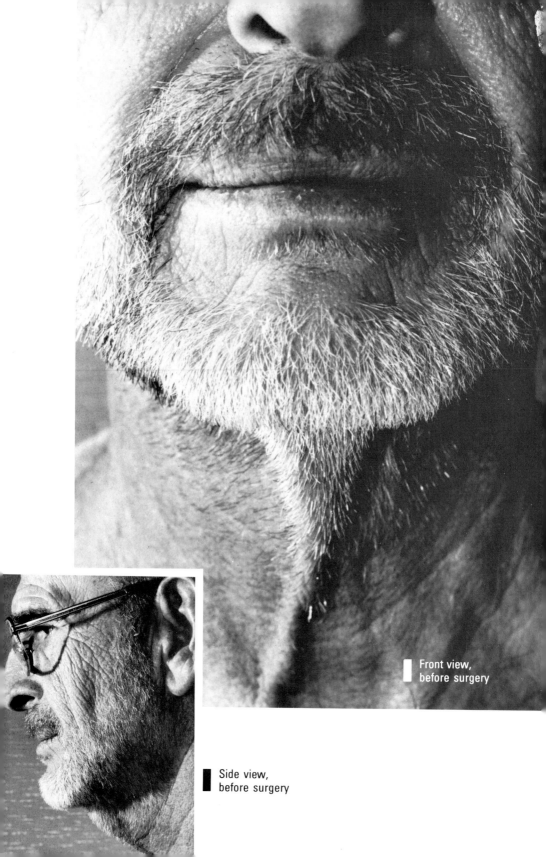

Front view,
before surgery

Side view,
before surgery

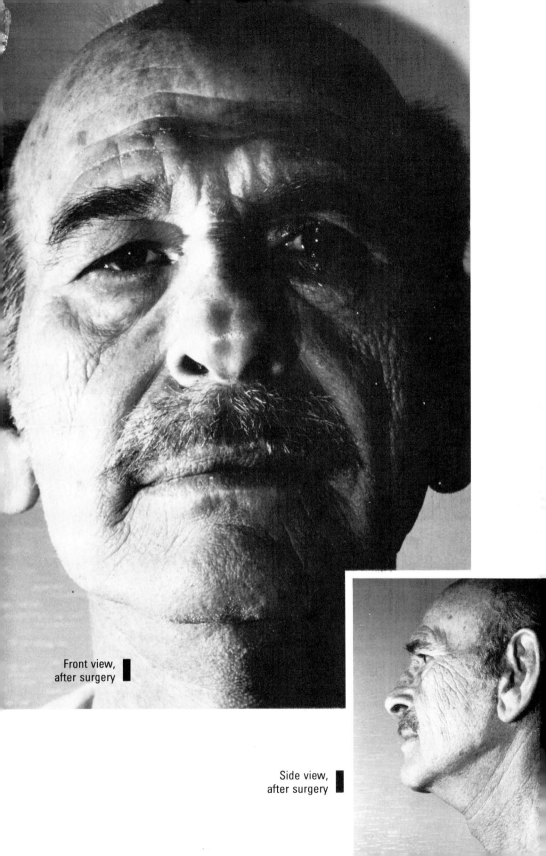

Front view,
after surgery

Side view,
after surgery

ear, so the male must remember to shave behind his ear after the operation.

In view of the scars resulting from a face-lift, the man's hairline must be taken into account. If the hairline is receding, or if there is a history of male pattern baldness in the family, special care must be taken to camouflage the scars. I advise all male patients to let their hair grow a little longer than usual before surgery so that it will hide the scars in the healing period following the operation.

Ears

Prominent ears are even more of an embarrassment to boys and men, since they cannot camouflage the problem with long hair as a girl can. The earlier the surgery is done, the better, in order to spare a young boy the sometimes unmerciful teasing of his peers. This surgery can also be done on older men who did not have the opportunity or the knowledge to repair the problem in youth. Incisions are usually concealed in the creases behind the ears, so this is one of the procedures having the least noticeable scars in plastic surgery.

Nose

Though the surgical approach to rhinoplasty is the same for men and women, the aesthetic ideal is different. For many, the male nose is a phallic symbol. It is traditionally left in larger proportion to the face in the male, even when a reduction is done.

Chins

Chins are often areas for which men request surgery. Modern males seem more concerned than females about a balanced profile, and a chin that is neither too small nor too large is considered by some to be a sign of masculinity. Some choose to hide defects with a beard or goatee; others elect surgery. The contour of a receding chin, which some consider to give an impression of weakness of character, may be built up with implants. An overprominent chin that may seem to give the appearance of belligerence can be pared down. One other cosmetic change sometimes requested is the addition of a dimple in the chin, a bit of adornment greatly admired by some women and one easily achieved with the surgeon's tools.

Breasts

Sometimes we forget that men are mammals and they, too, have breasts. Normally, they are small but some males develop *gynecomastia,* or prominent breasts. The causes of such development are varied, ranging from congenital problems to liver disease to hormonal imbalance. Sometimes young boys develop breasts at puberty, an embarrassment that makes them reluctant to expose their chests in the locker room or at the beach for fear of teasing.

As with the female, the procedure to correct this condition involves removal of some of the tissue responsible for the problem. Often this can be done with an incision around the nipple-areola area, so that the scar is easily camouflaged. If the condition is severe, however, more extensive incisions have to be made. Fortunately, hair on the chest helps to hide these scars for the male.

When the enlargement is due only to fatty tissue rather than excessive breast development, the treatment of choice is often lipolysis, which leaves only minimal scars.

Abdomen

Men who have lost a great deal of weight may find that the skin of the abdominal wall has become excessive, sometimes even producing an abdominal *panniculus,* or apron effect, a fold of skin that hangs all the way down to the thighs or knees. The excess skin need not actually hang down to cause the patient to have difficulty wearing clothing comfortably. He may also feel extremely uncomfortable about being seen in a bathing suit. The tummy tuck operation described in chapter 11 works well for such men. Excess skin and fat are removed, the muscle of the abdominal wall is strengthened if necessary, and the patient is left with a low scar in the pubic area, often hidden by the growth of hair in this region.

Thigh, buttock, arm

Body contouring is requested less frequently by men than by women, but some men also wish to rid themselves of abnormally large fat deposits in the thigh, buttock, or arm area, or in the lower back and shoulder regions. The procedures described in chapter 12 are the same for men. Lipolysis also is proving as effective for men as for women in removing fatty deposits with a minimal scar.

Hair

Despite the macho images of the shiny pates of Telly Savalas and the late Yul Brynner, baldness to most men signifies a loss of masculinity. Senator William Proxmire won sympathetic understanding from many men when he appeared on the Senate floor with the scars from his hair transplant operation still visible. Ninety-five percent of normal adult men will suffer some hair loss in the aging process, but like the senator, two out of five suffer an untimely loss caused by *male pattern alopecia* or baldness. The name comes from the fact that this type of baldness follows a definite pattern in the male. The hair usually recedes first in front, then grows sparse on top of the scalp, but remains healthy at the sides and back of the head. The process can begin as early as the twenties and thirties.

Seventy-five percent of adult women also suffer some hair loss, but it is usually diffuse rather than in a specific pattern.

These is some irony in the fact that many men consider a bald head a sign of lost virility, since it is actually a man's very maleness that helps to make him bald. In male pattern baldness, a hereditary condition, hair loss occurs because the hair follicles in certain areas are genetically predisposed to develop a sensitivity to the male hormone, androgen, and to stop producing hair. In fact, once a man is balding, there is only one known way to stop his hair from falling, and that is to rid him of his masculinity altogether. Eunuchs are never bald.

Not too long ago, nothing could be done for balding except to buy a toupee, but today there are two surgical procedures that can help.

One method is to use a metal tool to punch out small plugs of flesh from a donor site, a hair-bearing part of the scalp that is not threatened by alopecia, and transplant them in new sites in the bald area of the head that have been excavated with the same punch. Steady pressure with a surgical pad is usually enough to control bleeding following the transplant. A dressing is applied and the patient is taught how to remove it twenty-four hours after surgery. Antibiotics and a mild analgesic such as Tylenol with Codeine are given for two days after surgery. After a period of about three months, the hair begins to grow in its new site. Hair transplantation by the plug method results in individual tufts of hair rather than thick evenly distributed growth, but as long as hair continues to grow at the donor site, these transplanted hair plugs will last. Treatment of baldness by transplantation may also be done using strips of hair rather than plugs.

Another technique used for baldness works with *transposition flaps*. Unlike the methods just described where the plugs and strips used are cut off from their blood supply before

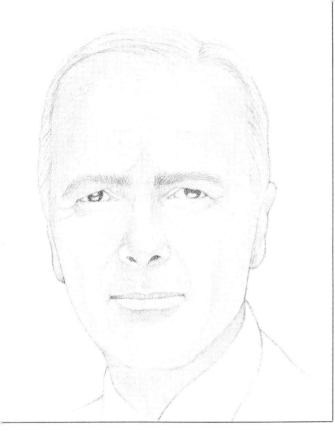

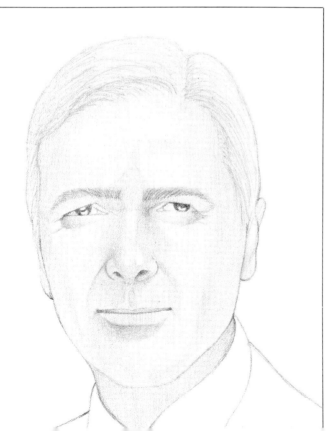

Hair transplants,
before and after

being transplanted, flaps retain their connection but are simply rotated into a new position. This was the primary treatment for male pattern baldness earlier in this century, and is coming back into prominence as the best way to restore the frontal hairline and to reduce baldness on the dome of the head in patients who still have enough hair to go around. Hair-bearing scalp is literally transposed or transferred from one area to another and the existing hair is rearranged. This method has the advantage of providing the natural density of hair follicles that cannot be reproduced in either plugs or strips. Hair flaps have the added advantage of permitting the surgeon greater leeway in providing for a normal direction of hair growth. The advisability, safety, and effectiveness of each method should be thoroughly discussed in consultations with a surgeon.

Recently a topical medication, minoxidil, has been introduced for the treatment of male pattern baldness. Minoxidil was initially used in the treatment of hypertension. It was noted, however, that when applied topically, a common effect is the growth of body hair. Therefore, it has been used to grow hair in 33⅓ percent of bald patients treated.

It was found to be exceptionally potent when taken orally because of its tendency to cause the body to retain fluids, therefore at present minoxidil is commonly used only in lotion form to treat baldness. The Upjohn Company undertook a pilot study to observe the effect of minoxidil applied to the scalp. Dr. Ronald Savin, associate clinical professor of dermatology at the Yale School of Medicine, one of the physicians involved in this study, states that minoxidil stopped hair loss in 95 percent of patients. It regrew hair sparsely in 70 percent, produced medium hair growth for 10 percent, and resulted in impressive growth for 3 to 5 percent. Dr. Savin also advises that it is most effective for hair loss at the crown of the head. At the present, minoxidil does not eliminate the need for surgical correction at the front area of the scalp. Using the two treatments together, however, may give the best overall result for patients with male pattern baldness. The Upjohn Company is currently seeking Federal Drug Administration approval for general use of the drug.

Tattoos and acne scars

One other request heard more frequently from males is the removal of tattoos. New methods to do this include the use of expansion devices, much like little balloons which are placed beneath the normal skin adjacent to the tattoo. Over the course of several weeks, this device is gradually filled with a saline solution. This causes the skin to expand, eventually permitting the excess stretched skin to be rotated over the defect created by the removal of the tattoo. The patient is left with a linear scar instead of the unaesthetic scar left by a skin graft. The expander also eliminates the need for a very large excision of skin involved by the tattoo. Usually a very tight closure is necessary and such closures run the risk of splitting open under stress.

Acne scars have already been mentioned in chapter 6, but it may be of some comfort for men to know that males were treated for this common affliction by abrasion methods centuries before modern man. The *Ebers Papyrus*, dating from around 1500 B.C., reveal that ancient Egyptian men were treated for acne scarring with an abrasive made from alabaster and grain. Where acne is concerned, the male beard is both a blessing and a bane—a blessing because it may be used to hide unsightly acne scars, but a bane because hair does not grow in scar tissue.

Not every male patient will emerge from cosmetic surgery looking like Michelangelo's *David*, or the Apollo Belvedere. But then seventeen-foot marble statues, even beautiful ones, are not the equal of a living, breathing male who is at peace with himself. If surgery can help the male regain a self-image that makes him feel more comfortable and confident, the plastic surgeon's mission has been accomplished.

IS COSMETIC SURGERY FOR YOU? 15

*I know of no more encouraging fact
than the unquestionable ability of
man to elevate his life by a
conscious endeavor.*

HENRY DAVID THOREAU

T hroughout history, men and women have been driven by
a basic human instinct to improve their natural appearance. In one era that meant painting and adorning the
face and body; today, for many hundreds of thousands
of people it means cosmetic surgery.

These are individuals who have decided to take action rather
than to endure things that make them unhappy about themselves every single day. They are taking advantage of the
greatly improved tools at the plastic surgeon's command to
correct defects and to slow the unwanted changes of time.

Is cosmetic surgery right for you, too? I hope this book has
helped you to answer that question by giving you a clearer
understanding of what is involved in each surgical procedure.

I thought it might be appropriate now to let you hear from a
few of my patients who can tell you first hand what cosmetic
surgery has meant to them. While I am changing the names to

protect their privacy, their comments are real, including their honest reactions to the healing period following surgery.

Jane O'Neill had a face-lift and her eyelids done at age fifty-two. "I thought about it for a couple of years," she says. "I had developed a double chin and lots of extra flesh around my neck that took away from my whole appearance. My face wasn't so wrinkled, but every time I looked in the mirror, it annoyed me. My husband said to me, 'Don't do it for me,' and a lot of friends asked, 'What are you doing that for? You don't need it.' But I wanted to do it for *myself* and *I* am very pleased with the outcome. It was uncomfortable right after surgery. My face didn't bruise but it was swollen. It took about three weeks before I wanted to be seen, and another few months before the stitches in front of the ear and the hairline faded, but I was able to cover them with my hair. Looking back, I feel there really wasn't much to it, the time passed quickly, and I'm happy every time I look in the mirror."

"I think turning forty had a lot to do with having nose surgery," states Carol Parker. "I guess it was time for my 'mid-life crisis' and I began thinking about doing what I had not done when I was younger. My spirits needed a lift and I finally had the courage to give myself that lift with surgery. My husband didn't say anything to discourage me, but my sixteen-year-old son was concerned. He told me, 'You don't need it,' and I think he was afraid it was going to make a big change in my looks. It didn't. I had a prominent nose with a bump on it. Surgery simply took away the bump, refined the shape, and made the nose a bit smaller, more in keeping with the rest of my features. It doesn't look like it was cosmetically repaired. It just looks nicer now. There was some discomfort the first couple of days when there was packing in the nose and I had to breathe through my mouth, but it was never overwhelming and once the packing came out it was fine. I'm a nurse, so I knew what to expect. My only regret is that I didn't do it years sooner."

At thirty-one, Maria Heller had lost weight and gotten into

shape by a regular exercise program, but she still had bulging thighs that did not respond to her efforts. "I felt I had lost enough weight and I didn't want to look emaciated, but I wanted my body to be in proportion," she explains. "When I heard about lipolysis, that seemed the perfect answer. Hearing about a good local doctor who did the procedure had a lot to do with making the decision to go ahead. Afterward it was painful for a day or two, but then it felt more or less like a bruise, like I had fallen. Truthfully, the worst of the operation was not pain but feeling dragged out from the anesthesia. But I couldn't afford to take time off from my job as a dental hygienist and I was back at work three days later and was able to function normally. The scars are small—about half an inch long on my inner knee and upper thigh—and they are fading nicely after three months. There is some rippling on the upper inner thigh, but that may fade also, and even if it doesn't, it is far better than the flab it replaced. I'm happy now whenever I put on jeans or tights. I took a lot of flack from my family about spending money on this, but I just figured I was giving myself the operation instead of buying clothes or a car. They can wait for next year. This was a present to myself."

It was a divorce and beginning to date that prompted Margie Anderson to want to get rid of the protruding stomach that was the result of her two pregnancies. "I was forty at the time, and my children said, 'Are you crazy?'" she recalls. "But it was something I wanted. My boyfriend didn't care, but I did. I looked like the Pillsbury doughboy, and my stomach was covered with stretch marks. I had a tummy tuck combined with lipolysis to take away the fat from the upper part of the abdomen near the waist. Now I can wear a bikini and it looks great. I had the operation four years ago, and I'm still pleased every time I look down and see my flat tummy.

"I never worried about the surgery once I made up my mind. I was medicated for the first day or so after surgery when it was still painful. Right afterward, you feel like you are never going to be able to move again, and then in three or four days it's suddenly okay and it keeps getting better and better each day. This is not a procedure that heals rapidly, but within six weeks I was back to myself, off on vacation and having a wonderful time. The healing of the incision from the tummy tuck hurt more than the lipolysis. The lipolysis area turned black and blue and felt like bruising, like when you fall down on the ice and bump yourself.

"Would I recommend it? Absolutely. In fact, I was so sold on plastic surgery that I went back two years ago to have my eyes done. That was a cinch, almost like having a tooth filled. I had the operation on Monday and on Thursday had twelve people over for Thanksgiving dinner."

Everyone has different motivation for having cosmetic surgery. What all of these patients had in common was a good mental attitude and a realistic view of what surgery could do for them. The purpose of cosmetic surgery is to make you look as good as it is possible for you to look. It cannot do more than that. If you are expecting a miraculous change, you will unquestionably be disappointed. It is not possible for any surgery to restore lost youth or change the basic structure of the body.

The aim of the surgeon is to have people say to you, "You look wonderful, refreshed, and rested. Have you been on vacation?" and not "Have you had plastic surgery?"

Nor is surgery an exact science. Some of the factors involved in producing the final result, including the healing process, are not entirely within the control of either the surgeon or the patient. It is impossible to absolutely guarantee results. How successful the surgery is and how much it enriches the lives of those who seek it depends on a combination of the patient's motivations and expectations, the competence of the surgeon, and always, the element of luck that protects the patient against unpredictable complications.

There are still many who ask whether it is worthwhile for a

basically healthy individual to take on the risks and scars of surgery for cosmetic reasons. Some see this only as vanity and have even asked me why a highly trained doctor would recommend what they see as nonessential surgery or use techniques such as lipolysis which break new medical ground.

When I am asked this question, I like to paraphrase an old Indian proverb that advises, "To understand the inner motivations of another being you must walk in his moccasins for a mile."

The 1980s version of that wisdom might advise us to sit in on a business meeting surrounded by younger people who are candidates for your job, or to look into the mirror at pouches, furrows, lines, and jowls that seem to grow by the day, marring an otherwise attractive face.

It might also suggest wearing designer jeans or form-fitting pants for a day—or perhaps an evening—with bulging thighs or tummy spoiling an otherwise attractive torso. This may be the only way truly to understand the embarrassment and trauma of the bearer of the bulge.

Psychologists consider taking action to improve the appearance and erase embarrassment as a highly positive step emotionally, a far cry from mere vanity. Dr. S. Michael Kalick of the University of Massachusetts notes that "literally hundreds of studies conducted in the past two decades corroborate the fact that attractiveness has a 'halo effect,' that we ascribe more positive characteristics to people we judge to be more attractive. This same bias influences our self-perception and, when we like ourselves better, others tend to respond to our own perceptions."

One wise and famous American thinker, Thomas Jefferson, defined happiness as "not being pained in body or troubled in mind." The reason that plastic surgeons perform cosmetic surgical procedures on otherwise healthy bodies is to restore peace of mind, an asset every bit as important as bodily health. When newer and more carefully tested surgical procedures promise better results with fewer scars, a conscientious surgeon will welcome them.

Not everyone is a candidate for plastic surgery. Some men and women take pride in the facial wrinkles and pouches that reflect their earthly experience. Others consider it neurotic to tamper with the body God has given them.

The final question is whether it is neurotic or psychologically healthy to want to look your best and to be good to yourself. Those thousands of well-adjusted persons who have been given an extra measure of happiness and self-confidence through plastic surgery would have no difficulty answering that question.

IMAGE ENHANCEMENT— SOME FINAL THOUGHTS

16

And if you do not find yourself beautiful yet, act as the creator of a state that is to be made beautiful: he cuts away here, he smooths there, he makes this line lighter, the other purer, until a lovely face has grown upon his work.

PLOTINUS, A.D. 270

In recent years, as I have talked to scores of women who come to consult me in order to improve their looks, I have come to realize that most people have two images of themselves: the person they see when they look in the mirror, and the ideal of who they would like to be.

Yes, it would be lovely to look like Sophia Loren or Cybill Shepherd, but most of us know that being a fashion model or a movie star is not a guarantee of happiness—and we also know that it isn't likely to happen to us. But all of us see room for self-improvement. The desire to realize our own best potential—to integrate the real self with the ideal—is a realistic goal that can be obtained through the concept I have come to call "Image Enhancement."

Image Enhancement means the development of the total person and personality so that the image one projects is not a false picture, but the enhanced true and best of our real selves.

As a surgeon, Image Enhancement is an integral part of the plastic surgery that I perform, not attempting to transform a person but to make the most of their own God-given assets. As with any procedure or process that alters the physical body, cosmetic surgery has a strong psychological impact and requires a total approach to helping the patient adjust to his or her new form or face.

Ideally, the surgery becomes only one step toward the goal of total enhancement, becoming the best one can possibly be in every way and achieving the special satisfaction and pride that comes with making ourselves better both physically and mentally.

Achieving this state of well-being means starting from the inside out, with proper nutrition and regular exercise to help you look and feel better every day. The skin reflects this healthy self-care with a clearer complexion and a healthier glow. The body responds by waking up to a new sense of fitness and well-being—and by trimming down, so that your clothing fits better and looks better on you.

In turn, the ego responds to your improved appearance with new self-confidence that inspires you to do justice to your new good looks. Proper makeup and hairstyling to show off your best features, clothing that makes the most of your figure's good points and minimizes the faults, colors that flatter your complexion—all of these are part of the total integrated concept of Image Enhancement.

Having seen the benefits to body and spirit these changes bring, I have added the concept of Image Enhancement to my offices in New York City and Waterbury, Connecticut, and have satellite centers in the Skin Care and Collagen Center at Cityplace in Hartford, Connecticut, and the Skin Care Center at the Spa located in the Fontainebleau Hotel in Miami, Florida. In each of these centers, I have enlisted the aid of consulting experts in the vital fields of exercise, nutrition, makeup, hairstyling, fashion, and color styling to bring their knowledge into a total program to help a woman bring out the very best in herself.

Plastic surgery can be an important part in your own Image Enhancement program, but with or without surgery, every woman can take steps to define her ideal self and work toward it. Each of us is our own greatest critic. Only if we begin to satisfy the demands we place on ourselves, to be all that we can be, will we gain the harmony of body, mind, and spirit, and the serenity, the confidence, and the security for a more fulfilling life.

ACKNOWLEDGMENTS

I t is not possible to record here a complete list of all the men and women who contributed so much to my education in becoming a plastic surgeon and the evolution of a happy and productive life.

My maternal grandparents, Erminia (Amelia) and Constant Gugiatti, who by word and deed provided me with so many good examples, the greatest of which was unselfish love. My paternal grandparents, Mary-Louise Callaghan and Timothy Moynahan, whom I never knew because of their early deaths, but whose influence was felt through the strength, courage, and general character of my father, who helped me so very much in becoming a doctor. My angel mother, whose patience, kindness, and love was so important and was always there. My only and older brother, Timothy Constant Moynahan, who has been best friend and confidant, as well as an example of excellence in every aspect of life. Mrs. G.

Scolese and Miss Ruth Hilding, grammar school teachers, who told their seven-year-old student they would be her patient when she became a doctor. Sister Suzanne O'Halloran, principal of Notre Dame Academy, for her encouragement and advice in selecting the right college for her sixth-grade pupil. James "Shimmer" Sheehan, father of my best friend, Helen Sheehan Winstead, for his kindness and generosity. The Sisters of Mercy at Sacred Heart High School. The dedicated Sisters of Charity at the College of Mount St. Vincent. My college roommate, Terry Ferrerio Petty, who burned so many midnight candles with me. The professors and physicians at the Medical College of Pennsylvania for the learning they imparted and the example they set. Those doctors, the majority of whom are surgeons, who inspired me to develop and perfect the art and science they so expertly and compassionately perform: Dr. Marcus Cox, Dr. Joseph Bergen, Dr. James Donaldson, Dr. Howard Kesseler, Dr. Charles McPeak, Dr. Peter Missier, Dr. Eugene Quash, and Dr. William Keavy. The chiefs of surgery whose departments it has been my privilege to be a part of since my internship to the present time: Dr. Walter Fischer, Dr. John O. Vieta, Dr. Edward Dunn, and Dr. Peter Fielding. Sister Margaret Rosita Kenney, Executive Director of St. Mary's Hospital, Waterbury, Connecticut, who was beginning her career in nursing when I was born at St. Mary's, and who was chief administrator when I was appointed to the attending staff years later. Kathleen McGrory, President of Hartford College for Women, who collaborated with me on the writing of this book. Eleanor Berman, who also greatly assisted in the production of the final manuscript. Anne Akers, friend and associate, whose efforts resulted in the publishing of this book. Edna Dufresne and Susan Melchior, R.N., who retyped the preceding pages until they were right. Laraine Colaci Primini, R.N., Patricia Miller, L.P.N., and Gail Guerriero, R.N., dedicated nurses who take such good care of those patients of mine who place their well-being in our hands. Other members of my staff: Mary Clifford, Lucille Ortelle, Dr. Louissa Pirnia, Annemarie Callinicos, Channie Blanchfield, Corinne Rabtoy, Judy Hicks, R.N., and Teanie Trottman, all of whom have been so kind and good to those people I have taken care of. Tammy Aronson, C.R.N.A., talented nurse and anesthetist, who has devoted great time and effort to the care and well-being of my patients. All the dedicated doctors and nurses who have joined their lives with mine in caring for those people whose lives are so important to us.

INDEX